ENDOCRINOLOGY RESEARCH AND CLINICAL DEVELOPMENTS

THYROID NODULES

RISK FACTORS, DIAGNOSIS AND MANAGEMENT

Endocrinology Research and Clinical Developments

Additional books in this series can be found on Nova's website under the Series tab.

Additional e-books in this series can be found on Nova's website under the e-book tab.

ENDOCRINOLOGY RESEARCH AND CLINICAL DEVELOPMENTS

THYROID NODULES

RISK FACTORS, DIAGNOSIS AND MANAGEMENT

MARSHA VASQUEZ
EDITOR

NOVA BIOMEDICAL
New York

Library of Congress Cataloging-in-Publication Data

ISBN: 978-1-63483-592-3

Library of Congress Control Number: 2015947574

Published by Nova Science Publishers, Inc. † New York

Contents

Preface

Thyroid nodules are commonly diagnosed in adults, although they are rare in children affecting only 1%-2% of this population. Since the late 1960's, ultrasound (US) has become essential in the examination of the thyroid gland as a non-invasive, rapid and easily reproducible imaging study. This book provides the reader with a framework from which to develop a differential diagnosis, risk factors and evaluation plan for both children and adults presented with thyroid nodules. Risk factors and management of a thyroidectomy are presented as well, and the challenges it poses for the surgeon who undertakes endocrine surgery. The final chapter evaluates the association between Hashimoto's thyroiditis and differentiated thyroid cancer.

Chapter I – Thyroid nodules are commonly diagnosed in adults, while they are rare in children affecting only 1%–2% of this population based on clinical examination. This pathologic condition is rare and requires investigation because the incidence of malignancy is higher than in adults. After evaluation of the medical history and detailed physical examination, the second step is an assessment of thyroid function and measurement of calcitonin level. Ultrasonography (USG) is an easily applicable, noninvasive method that provides maximum benefit in the diagnostic and management approach. Fine-needle aspiration (FNA) biopsy guided by the results of USG has 90% accuracy and is very useful in the selection of patients for surgery. The objective of this chapter is to discuss the epidemiology, medical history, physical examination, laboratory and imaging methods with the diagnosis and therapeutic approaches of nodular thyroid disease in the pediatric population.

Chapter II – Since the late 1960's, ultrasound (US) has become essential in the examination of the thyroid gland with the increased availability of high-frequency linear array transducers and computer-enhanced imaging capabilities in a clinic-based setting. As a non-invasive, rapid and easily reproducible imaging study, US has a broadened utility beyond the simple confirmation of thyroid nodules and their size. Clinic-based US can image thyroid lesions and provide additional information in real time with greater clarity that otherwise might have been missed by history and physical examination. The routine use of diagnostic imaging has led to the incidental discovery of many non-palpable thyroid nodules, most of which require further evaluation and management. Specifically, US has become useful in the qualitative analysis and delineation of such thyroid nodules based on features for malignancy or benignity. Furthermore, examination of cervical lymph node basins for staging purposes and characterization of the contralateral thyroid lobe are also achievable with clinic-based US, which may influence the extent of the intended thyroid operation. Additionally, US-guided fine-needle aspiration can be crucial in the preoperative investigation of a thyroid nodule. It provides accurate cytologic sampling from thyroid nodules thereby minimizing inconclusive specimens. This chapter discusses the role and utility of clinic-based US in the evaluation and management of thyroid nodules.

Chapter III – While thyroid carcinoma is rare in the pediatric and adolescent population, it is important for pediatricians and other health care providers to assess for risk of malignancy and order appropriate diagnostic tests in conjunction with consultation with an endocrinologist when confronted with a thyroid mass in a young patient. This chapter will provide the reader with a framework from which to develop a differential diagnosis and initial evaluation plan for such a child or adolescent presenting with a thyroid nodule; identify the risk factors associated with malignant thyroid nodules; appreciate the limitations of ultrasonography and fine-needle aspiration biopsy in the assessment of a thyroid nodule; recognize the risk factors inherent in surgical thyroidectomy; and understand the role of radio-active iodine treatment in the management of thyroid carcinoma. General pediatricians, sub-specialists, and parents alike will welcome the summary of the current state of knowledge in the management of pediatric thyroid nodules and well differentiated thyroid carcinoma (WDTC).

Chapter IV – In the last decade, the incidence of malignant thyroid cancer has increased worldwide. This escalation has derived either from a precocious individualization of small carcinomas or a major occurrence of large carcinomas. As a counterweight to early diagnosis, the mortality has not decreased but has rather increased. Epithelial malignant cancers of the thyroid emerge as nodules set up by two different cellular types such as follicular and parafollicular cells, namely C cells. The former, producing thyroid hormones, develop either well differenced thyroid carcinomas (WDTC) or anaplastic carcinomas; while the latter, secreting calcitonin, make up medullary thyroid carcinomas (MTC). WDTC account for 90% of all thyroid cancers and are classified as papillary thyroid cancer (PTC) (80–85%), follicular thyroid cancer (FTC) (10–15%) and Hurtle cell carcinoma (HCC) (3–5%). Overall, WDTC have good prognosis with disease free survival close to 95% for PTC and 80% for FTC. ATC are occurring in 1 to 2% of thyroid cancers and display a poor prognosis. MTC include the remaining 5 to 9% of thyroid cancer and show a relatively poor prognosis. Multiple gene mutations and rearrangements harbour in thyroid cancers. Affected genes include RET, BRAF, PI3KCA, RAS, MET and Galectin. Chromosomal rearrangements involve especially chromosome 7 and 10. Morphology of cells already plays a main role for identification of cancer in nodules and to drive patients toward appropriate treatments. The latest is that molecular medicine may work in diagnostic identification of thyroid cancers as a marker and therefore, could modify the flow chart for management of thyroid nodules.

Chapter V – The medullary thyroid carcinoma (MTC) is developed from thyroid C cells that secrete calcitonin (CT). MTC accounts for 5–10% of thyroid cancers with a 1–2% incidence in nodular thyroid diseases. It is sporadic in the majority of cases and familial in 20 to 30% of cases. Familial hereditary form is a result of a germline mutation in the *RET* proto-oncogene and can be seen in familial medullary thyroid cancer (FMTC) or as part of the multiple endocrine neoplasia (MEN) syndrome type 2 (2A or 2B). MTC is frequently solitary nodule which is often associated with nodal metastasis. Confirmation is obtained by a high basal calcitonin level which represents specific biological marker. Surgery is the only curative treatment and should consist of total thyroidectomy with central and ipsilateral or bilateral lateral lymph node dissection. A prophylactic thyroidectomy may be performed for at-risk members in the familial form. Radiation therapy does not currently play a significant role in the treatment of MTC. For locally advanced or metastatic MTC, chemotherapy provides little benefit. RET target gene therapy (mainly tyrosine kinase inhibitors) appears as possible promise therapeutic for the future. The prognosis of MTC depends on both the stage of the disease and the extent of the initial surgery.

Chapter VI – Thyroidectomy is a relatively common procedure and like any surgery procedure involves risks. Thyroidectomy poses many challenges for the surgeon who undertakes endocrine surgery. Fatal complications are rare, but the incidence of minor complications and their sequelae are common. The recurrent laryngeal nerve injury and hypocalcemia due to hypoparathyroidism are the most common early complications after a thyroid operation. Hypocalcemia is generally transient, but it may be permanent requiring lifelong administration of calcium plus vitamin D. Unilateral recurrent laryngeal nerve injury results in hoarseness or dysphonia due to laryngeal paralysis with unilateral vocal cord immobility. Bilateral recurrent laryngeal nerve palsy results in dramatic symptoms of acute life-threatening dyspnea. Other complications of thyroid surgery include postoperative hemorrhage, seroma, hematoma, respiratory obstruction, wound infection and sepsis. Risk factors of most complications should be considered before surgery. In this chapter, we propose to study the complications of thyroidectomy as well as risk factors and current treatment modalities based on an evaluation of the recent studies of morbidity.

Chapter VII – The association between Hashimoto's thyroiditis and differentiated thyroid cancer has been discussed in literature, but the relationship is still controversial. Coexistence of these two diseases is reported in up to 30% of cases, suggesting that there might be a pathological and causative link between them. On the other hand, the presence of thyroiditis may indicate a lower recurrence rate and a better prognosis of thyroid cancer. The diagnosis and follow-up in these cases may be challenging even for experts and require a wide range of laboratory, ultrasound (US), and morphology criteria in addition to an individualized approach. In the background of Hashimoto's thyroiditis with the typical heterogeneous echotexture with hypoechoic micronodules and hypervascularity, the sonographic appearance of a focal thyroid lesion may vary greatly, making it more difficult to differentiate between benign and malignant nodules, as well as between true nodules and pseudonodules. Fine needle aspiration biopsy is currently the best diagnostic test for the preoperative evaluation of thyroid nodules, including those coexistent with thyroiditis. However, the presence of lymphocytes and Hürthle cells may represent a potential source of error in cytological interpretation. Furthermore, there is an overlap in immunohistochemical staining and molecular profile between papillary carcinoma and Hashimoto's thyroiditis. The aim of the present review is to summarize available evidence for the link between Hashimoto's thyroiditis and differentiated thyroid cancer with emphasis on US and cytology interpretation, the role of US elastography, and molecular markers. The promising use of thyroglobulin antibodies (TgAb) for postoperative monitoring of these patients will also be discussed.

In: Thyroid Nodules
Editor: Marsha Vasquez

ISBN: 978-1-63483-592-3

Chapter I

Thyroid Nodules in Children

Moncef Sellami**, Souha Kallel, Mohamed Masmoudi, Ilhem Charfeddine, Malek Mnejja and Abdelmonem Ghorbel

Department of otorhinolaryngology-Head and Neck Surgery
Habib Bourguiba University Hospital,
Sfax, Tunisia

Abstract

Thyroid nodules are commonly diagnosed in adults, while they are rare in children affecting only 1%-2% of this population based on clinical examination.

This pathologic condition is rare and requires investigation because the incidence of malignancy is higher than in adults.

After evaluation of the medical history and detailed physical examination, the second step is an assessment of thyroid function and measurement of calcitonin level.

Ultrasonography (USG) is an easily applicable, noninvasive method that provides maximum benefit in the diagnostic and management approach.

* Phone: +21624050980. E-mail: sellami_moncef@yahoo.fr

Fine-needle aspiration (FNA) biopsy guided by the results of USG has 90% accuracy and is very useful in the selection of patients for surgery.

The objective of this chapter is to discuss the epidemiology, medical history, physical examination, laboratory and imaging methods with the diagnosis and therapeutic approaches of nodular thyroid disease in the pediatric population.

Introduction

Thyroid nodules are commonly diagnosed in adults, although they are rare in pediatrics (<18 years of age), affecting only 1%–2% of this population based on clinical examination [1, 2].

Among 175 consecutive children requiring thyroid surgery at Children's Hospital Boston, thyroid nodules were, by far, the most common indication (83%), followed by hyperthyroidism (7%) and goiter (7%) [3].

Exposure to ionizing radiations is another well-known risk factor for thyroid cancer, especially for papillary carcinoma [4].

Approximately 5% of adult nodules are malignant and 25% of pediatric nodules are malignant [5]. Children with thyroid cancer present at a more advanced stage of disease than do adults with a higher incidence of lymphadenopathy and pulmonary metastases but a lower mortality rate than do adults [6]. Thyroid nodular disease in children requires a detailed clinical examination comprised of prior history of thyroid disease in the patient or in their family, history of radiation exposure, careful palpation of the thyroid and lymph nodes, blood tests, ultrasonography, and cytological assessment [2].

For pediatric thyroidectomy and thyroid lobectomy, a collaboration of high-volume endocrine and pediatric surgeons, as well as pediatric endocrinologists at a dedicated pediatric medical center provides optimal surgical outcomes [7].

Epidemiology

Incidence and Prevalence

The prevalence of nodules in adults ranges from about 5% by a physical examination to up to 35% by ultrasound scan and up to 65% in autopsy studies. However, there is limited knowledge of the prevalence of thyroid nodules in the pediatric population [8].

The reported incidence of thyroid nodules in children and adolescents is estimated to be between 1% and 2% [1]. However, this incidence may be increasing because diagnostic radiological procedures are detecting incidental thyroid nodules [9].

The prevalence of thyroid nodules detected by palpation ranged from 2.2 to 15 per 1000 subjects in children [10, 11].

Although the incidence of thyroid disease is relatively small in children, the proportion of cases that are malignant is significantly greater when compared with adult [7]. When compared to adults, children have four times greater risk of malignancy when a thyroid nodule is diagnosed [12].

Age Distribution

Thyroid nodules are uncommon in children and the peak incidence of thyroid cancer occurs in children from 10 to 18 years of age [13].

The incidence of thyroid cancer seems to increase with age. In a study of 235 children and adolescents who followed Maria Skłodowska Memorial Cancer Center and Institute of Oncology for thyroid cancer, 5% were diagnosed under 6 years old, 10% with 7–9 years, increasing substantially after 10 years old [12].

Sex Predilection

Thyroid cancer in children has a predilection for female patients [12].

Focusing on the majority of children who underwent thyroid surgery at the Children's Hospital Boston from 1970 to 2004, Scholz et al. [3]. observed a strong sex predominance with a 3.7:1 female to male ratio. This ratio decreased markedly to 1.25:1 (15 females vs 12 males) in children younger than 10 years.

Ethnic Distribution

Thyroid cancer is more common in whites compared with African Americans [14].

Risk Factors

Radiation

Previous radiation is related to a higher incidence of thyroid cancer in a dose-dependent manner, especially for papillary carcinoma [15]. Children's thyroid gland is much more sensitive to the carcinogenic effects of ionizing radiation than that of adults.

Lower doses than those observed for most other radiation-induced cancers may induce thyroid carcinogenesis (to the order of 0.10 Gy). While high doses (>30 Gy) result in a lowered risk of thyroid cancer, probably due to cell killing [16]. In the past 60 years, the incidence of thyroid carcinoma in the pediatric age group presented two distinct peaks [12].

The first occurred around 1950 due to the use of radiation for the treatment of common childhood conditions such as Tinea capitis, acne, chronic tonsillitis, and thymus hyperplasia [17].

In these cases, the thyroid carcinoma was diagnosed on average 10–20 years after exposure, but with risk persisting until 40 years later. The thyroid gland in children has one of the highest risk coefficients of any organ and is the only tissue with convincing evidence for risk about 1.10 Gy [17]. These data led to the acceptance of ionizing radiation as a risk factor for the development of thyroid cancer [18].

Studies of children treated with ionizing radiation for a variety of benign and malignant diseases have demonstrated that doses as low as 0.10 Gy or as high as 60 Gy can induce thyroid tumors [19]. A second peak incidence occurred in the 1990s in some regions of Eastern Europe on behalf of the nuclear accident that occurred in Chernobyl in 1986 (ie Belarus). Children exposed to the Chernobyl accident at an age up to 10 years were at high risk for thyroid cancer [20, 21].

A papillary cancer was typically present in these patients. Radiation treatment to the head, neck, and upper chest for treatment of other childhood malignancies has been associated with the development of a secondary thyroid malignancy.

The risk of thyroid cancer increases in proportion to increasing radiation doses up to 20 to 29 Gy but then decreases with higher doses [14, 16]. Furthermore, it should be considered that there is increasing evidence that chemotherapy might also be a causative factor [22].

Prior Malignancy

As a complication after treatment for a primary malignancy, thyroid cancer constitutes 9% of secondary malignancies [23]. Hodgkin's lymphoma is the most common malignancy associated with subsequent thyroid cancer.

Age

Pediatric thyroid nodules behave differently than adult nodules. The rate of malignancy in pediatric nodules may be as high as 25% compared with the rate of 5% in adult nodules [14]. In the pediatric population, children under 10 years with thyroid nodule are at higher risk of cancer [5, 24].

Genetic

Various genetic events may account for the disparity in behavior of the different histologic subtypes of thyroid cancer:

1. Genetic alterations such as RET/TRK rearrangements or BRAF and RAS mutations usually lead to signaling derangements in the mitogen-activated protein kinase pathway [4].
2. RAS protooncogene mutations usually lead to signaling derangements in the mitogen-activated protein kinase pathway. RAS proto-oncogene mutations are found in 20% of papillary cancers and 80% of follicular cancers [25].
3. Several types of rearrangement known to occur in thyroid cancer, including RET/PTC, NTRK1 and BRAF/AKAP9, are more common are found predominantly in radiation-induced papillary thyroid carcinoma [26]
4. RET genetic translocations can be detected in 35% of papillary thyroid cancers [27]. RET mutations are more known for their role in the medullary thyroid carcinoma (MTC) [4].
5. Additional genetic mutations in the v-Raf (Virus-induced rapidly accelerated fibrosarcoma) murine sarcoma viral oncogene homolog B1 (BRAF) oncogene are also associated with papillary cancer. This mutation has a low prevalence in children compared with adults [28]

6. In follicular carcinomas, genetic alterations commonly consist of PAX8-PPAR gamma translocations or RAS mutations. CTNNB1 and p53 mutations have been implicated in the development of anaplastic carcinomas [29].

Thyroid Nodule and Cancer-Related Inherited Conditions

Familial conditions that may be associated with thyroid nodules and malignancy are listed in Table 1 [14]. We should be aware of these genetic syndromes presenting or associated with thyroid nodules, most of which are overgrowth, hamartomatous, and cancer predisposition syndromes with a preponderance of non-thyroidal tumors [4].

Table 1. Syndromes and inheritable conditions associated with thyroid nodules and cancer

	Gene Involved	Features
Cowden	PTEN tumor suppressor	Thyroid, GI, breast, uterine tumors
Familial adenomatous polyposis	APC gene (AD)	Increased risk of thyroid cancer, GI polyps with increased risk of malignant transformation
Gardner	APC gene (AD)	Increased risk thyroid cancer, jaw osteomas, GI polyps with increased risk of malignant transformation
Peutz-Jeghers	STK11 gene (AD)	Increased risk thyroid cancer, jaw osteomas, GI polyps with increased risk of malignant transformation
MEN 2A	RET proto-oncogene (AD)	Medullary thyroid carcinoma, pheochromocytoma, parathyroid
MEN 2B	RET proto-oncogene (AD)	Medullary thyroid carcinoma, pheochromocytoma, mucosal neuromas, Marfanoid

AD, autosomal dominant, GI, gastrointestinal.

Pathology

- The pathological classification of cancers in children is based on standard definitions set by the World Health Organization (WHO), with histological criteria the same for children and adults [30].
- Pediatric thyroid malignancies are nearly all well-differentiated subtypes of papillary, follicular, and medullary. Anaplastic carcinoma

is typically seen in older adults. Children present at a more advanced stage of disease than do adults and with a higher incidence of lymphadenopathy and pulmonary metastases [14, 13, 31].

- In a study including all malignant neoplasms of the thyroid gland, registered between 1978 and 1997 in 61 European cancer registries (1690 cases) five histological groups were considered. The large majority of the thyroid cancers were papillary (75%), the remainder was composed of follicular (13%), medullary (8%), 'other' carcinomas (3.6%) and of anaplastic type (0.4%) [32].
- Papillary thyroid cancer is frequently multicentric and tend to spread via lymphatics to regional nodes. Metastases to lung and bone are usually very late findings. Pathologically, psammoma bodies are seen and there is usually a prominent follicular pattern [13].
- Follicular thyroid cancer (FTC) is less common and is difficult pathologically to differentiate from normal thyroid tissue or follicular adenoma [13]. They are typically unifocal tumors and more prone to metastasize hematogenously (bone, liver, and lung) [13]. Histologic variants of FTC include: Hürthle cell, clear cell, and insular carcinoma [30]
- Medullary thyroid carcinoma originates from parafollicular C cells. MTC may arise spontaneously or in association with familial medullary thyroid carcinoma, multiple endocrine neoplasia (MEN)IIA, or IIB syndromes [13].

Clinical Presentation

Initial evaluation should include a thorough history and physical examination.

History

Medical History

Other concomitant thyroid diseases (autoimmune thyroid disease, thyroid dysgenesis, dyshormonogenesis), the environment (iodine deficiency region), previous cancer, neck radiation therapy should be questioned in the history.

History of radiotherapy to the neck and previous cancers are also risk factors for the development of malignancy.

The Family History

A family history of thyroid neoplasms or of inherited condition or syndromes that are associated with thyroid cancer are important risk factors for the development of pediatric thyroid cancer [14].

Roy et al. [33] found a positive history of thyroid cancer in the family in 26.4% of the cases with malignancy in a retrospective analysis of 207 children who underwent total thyroidectomy, and such a positive history increased (1.4 times) the risk of malignancy.

Symptoms

Most pediatric patients with differentiated thyroid cancer present with an asymptomatic, incidentally noted solitary neck mass due to a thyroid nodule. Patient can have variable states of thyroid function: euthyroid, hypothyroid, or hyperthyroid [14].

The clinician is expected to look for dysphagia, dysphonia, shortness of breath to assess local compression, and for tachycardia, increased differential pressure, hyperhydrosis, diarrhea, weight loss, increased appetite, heat intolerance, tremors, or exophthalmia for hyperthyroidism [4].

Physical Examination

A complete physical examination with special attention to the thyroid gland and any cervical mass is important.

The nodule limits, fixation to surrounding tissue, sensitivity, should be evaluated in detail on the physical examination. The probability of malignancy is higher in nodules that are non-tender, have irregular borders, are fixed to the surrounding tissue, and are accompanied by regional lymphadenopathy [34] [35]. The finding of lymph node enlargement is of crucial importance. Hard and firm lymph nodes are commonly considered highly suggestive of thyroid malignancy [4].

Lymph nodes involvement at diagnosis is present in 40–80% of children with differentiated thyroid cancer, compared with a 20–50% incidence in adults [2, 25].

In hereditary cases, MTC is generally multicentric and bilateral [36].

A physical examination should be complete and extensive and should aim to detect signs and dysmorphisms typical of syndromes associated with thyroid nodules [4].

Diagnostic procedures

Laboratory Data

The main purposes of laboratory assays are to evaluate thyroid function and to assess calcitonin secretion.

Serum Thyroid-Stimulating Hormone (TSH)

Determinations of thyroid-stimulating hormone (TSH) level at diagnosis is mandatory to assess thyroid function and establish the further workup.

If the TSH is suppressed, indicating a hyperfunctioning nodule, a radionuclide scan (scintigraphy) should be performed. If the TSH is not suppressed, a thyroid ultrasound (US) should be performed [37]. Hyperthyroidism is commonly caused by a toxic adenoma with a prevalence ranging from 0.7 to 5% [38]. Recently, there has been much interest for TSH determinations in nodule diagnosis [4]. Because cases with malignant nodules are most likely seen in the upper normal serum TSH range (> 2.8 mU/L), serum TSH concentration can serve as a predictor of thyroid cancer in pediatric patients with thyroid nodules and can inform the decision of when to submit patients to further investigation by cytology [39].

Calcitonin

Routine assessment of calcitonin levels is mandatory in patients with a suspicion of familial MTC, MEN2, and in cases showing a cytology suggestive of medullary neoplasm [4].

Since 2006, The European Thyroid Association recommended the determination of calcitonin in the initial diagnostic evaluation of thyroid nodules because it proved its value in finding medullary carcinoma at an earlier stage [40].

Corrias et al. recommend a systematic evaluation of calcitonin levels in pediatric patients [4].

However in the recent Revised American Thyroid Association Guidelines for the Management of Medullary Thyroid Carcinoma (2015) opinions of experts diverged regarding the usefulness of measuring serum calcitonin levels in patients with nodular goiters, the Task Force recommended that physicians decide whether the technique is useful in the management of patients in their clinic [41].

A basal calcitonin level over 100 pg/ml is considered significant for medullary thyroid cancer [35].

Other Laboratory Data

- Serum parathyroid hormone, calcium and vitamin D measurements should be performed to evaluate the calcium metabolism.
- Measurements of thyroid autoantibodies (particularly anti-antibodies thyroid peroxidase (AbTPO) are useful for the detection of autoimmune thyroiditis but their contribution to the differential diagnosis of thyroid nodules is poor [40].
- Measurement of serum thyroglobulin (Tg) has no role in the diagnostic evaluation of thyroid nodules, since its concentration is correlated with the size rather than with the nature of the nodule or of the thyroid gland [42].
- Assays in the washout fluid from FNAB of cervical lymph nodes:
    - The thyroglobulin measurement in the needle washout after fine-needle aspiration has been reported to increase the sensitivity of FNA in identifying lymph node metastases from differentiated thyroid cancer [43].
    - Calcitonin measurement in fine-needle aspirate washouts examination for diagnosis of primary or metastatic medullary thyroid carcinoma is particularly useful in the presence of non-diagnostic FNA [44].

Imaging Evaluation

Ultrasonography (USG)

Thyroid USG is inexpensive, radiation free, quick procedure, and requires no sedation in children. USG should be performed in all patients with thyroid nodules [14].

USG is a real-time imaging test that has become an integral part of the physical exam for evaluating thyroid nodules in patients under 21 years of age [45].

The USG report should include information on the location, composition (solid, cystic, mixed), echogenicity, halo sign of the nodule(s), calcification (microcalcification, macrocalcification, peripheral (eggshell) calcification), boundaries (regular, irregular), length/width ratio, and Doppler findings (blood flow within the nodules) [35].

The criteria for suspected malignancy are summarized in Table 2 [5]

Table 2. Ultrasonography Findings Indicating Malignancy

Solitary solid lesion
Hypoechogenicity
Subcapsular localization
Irregular margins of the lesion
Invasive growth (no compression of adjacent tissues)
Heterogenous nature of the lesion
Multifocal lesions within an otherwise clinically solitary nodule
Microcalcifications
High intranodular flow by Doppler (with normal TSH)
Suspicious regional lymph nodes accompanying thyroid nodule

Ultrasound elastography is a new technique that has been used to acquire information on tissue stiffness noninvasively in recent years. It has good diagnostic efficacy for differentiation of benign and malignant thyroid nodules in adults. Elastography can be used as a supplementary tool with sonography and can potentially reduce unnecessary fine-needle-aspiration biopsy [46].

To date, there are no data regarding the use of elastography in pediatric thyroid nodules.

Scintigraphy

Technetium Tc 99 m, iodohippurate sodium I 131, or sodium iodide I 123 scintigraphy can detect ectopic thyroid tissue and also help confirm the absence of thyroid tissue in the normal location [47].

If the TSH is suppressed, scintigraphy can confirm an independently active nodule [48].

Scintigraphy is not routinely used and has few indications (described above).

Fine-Needle Aspiration (FNA)

Fine-needle aspiration (FNA) plays an essential role in the evaluation of patients with a thyroid nodule. In a prospective study, concerning 75 patients under 19 years of age with thyroid nodules, the FNA results showed a positive predictive value (PPV) and negative predictive value (NPV) for malignancy of 75% and 92%, respectively, with sensitivity of 75%, specificity 92%, and diagnostic efficiency of 89% [49].

Ultrasound FNA of thyroid nodules in children and adolescents is highly accurate in experienced hands. With the Ultrasound FNA of 52 pediatric thyroid nodules, Izquierdo et al. [1] found a sensitivity of 100%, a specificity of 88.9% without any false-negatives but they found one false positive case. The overall cytological diagnostic accuracy was 93.7% [1]. These results were superior to those of FNA done by palpation previously published by the same team [50] where sensitivity, specificity and accuracy were respectively 63%, 58,3% and 11,2%.

The 2015 ATA pediatric guidelines recommends that all FNA in children should be performed under USG-guidance [51].

FNA improves the selection of pediatric patients requiring surgery, and patients with a benign cytological diagnosis can be safely followed clinically [1].

The Bethesda System for Reporting Thyroid Cytopathology (a guideline for the interpretation of FNA cytology) have been set forth in the adult population [52]. The Bethesda criteria comprise six classes, where each class has an implied cancer risk which can help guide surgical decision making (Table 3).

Table 3. FNA categories under the Bethesda classification, malignancy risk in adults and ATA management guidelines [37, 53]

Bethesda criteria	Malignancy risk (%)	Management
I Nondiagnostic I	1–4	Repeat US guided FNA [a]
II Benign	0–3	Clinical follow-up
III AUS/FLUS	5–15	Repeat FNA [a] or lobectomy
IV Suspicious for follicular neoplasm	15–30	Lobectomy
V Suspicious for malignancy	60–75	Lobectomy or total thyroidectomy
VI Malignant	97–99	Total thyroidectomy

A: If repeat FNA yields the same result, consider lobectomy. ATA; American Thyroid Association, FNA; fine needle aspiration, AUS; atypia of undetermined significance, FLUS; follicular lesion of undetermined significance

Although the malignancy risk for each Bethesda class is not well studied in children, the American Thyroid Association guidelines promote the same management for each Bethesda class for children and adults [53, 37].

Compared to the adult, pediatric thyroid nodules have an increased risk of malignancy and the implied cancer risk for each Bethesda category is most likely different [54]. In a recent study Including Fifty-six patients (66 nodules) under 18 years showed that the proportion of nodules with malignancy for BI-BVI was: 0%, 0%, 18%, 100%, 100% and 100% [53].

Indication of FNA in pediatric thyroid nodules are [14]:

- All pediatric solid thyroid nodules greater than 1 cm in diameter
- Nodules that are between 0.5 cm and 1 cm should be biopsied by FNA if any other historical, physical examination, or ultrasonographic risk factors is found.

Molecular Genetic Studies with FNA

Recently, many molecular markers have been investigated in an attempt to increase diagnostic accuracy of indeterminate fine needle aspiration cytology

(Bethesda III) and to avoid unnecessary complications and costs associated with thyroid surgery [55, 56].

The following genes carry somatic mutations in differentiated thyroid cancer and have been studied as potential tools to enhance the diagnostic accuracy of indeterminate FNA lesions – either alone or in combination as a panel [56]:

- BRAF
- RET-PTC
- RAS
- PAX8/PPAR-γ

Although no pediatric studies exist regarding these assays, emerging studies in adults may shed light on their utility [15, 51].

Miscellaneous Conditions

Nonpalpable Thyroid Nodules

Nonpalpable thyroid nodules appear to be of less importance in children and adolescents than in adults [5]

Palpable and nonpalpable pediatric nodules have a similar risk of malignancy and a common diagnostic approach should be used. Thus, Corrias et al. [57] opt for FNA whenever a nodule is accidentally revealed by ultrasound .

Thyroglossal Cyst and the Risk of Cancer

Thyroglossal duct cyst arises from remnants of the embryologic thyroglossal duct, is the most common developmental anomalies present during thyroid development [58, 59].

The occurence of carcinoma within the cyst or tract is very rare (less than 1% of cases) [58].

Pfeiffer et al. have reported that from the 26 cases of pediatric patients with thyroglossal cyst carcinoma in English literature 21 were papillary carcinoma, 3 mixed papillary-follicular and 1 patient had no pathology information [59].

Management of thyroglossal duct carcinoma should be similar to that of differentiated thyroid cancer and based on risk group stratification [58].

Ectopic Thyroid

Ectopic thyroid tissue can be found in sites along the descent of the thyroglossal duct, with the most common site (90%) being the lingual region [14, 60].

Although the lingual thyroid is in most cases asymptomatic, it can cause dysphagia, hemoptysis, or airway obstruction in some patients [14, 61].

This condition may be clinically suspected when examination reveals the presence of a median basi lingual mass [62].

Diagnostic management of thyroid ectopy is performed by radionuclide thyroid imaging, ultrasonography, CT scan, MRI, biopsy and thyroid function tests [62].

The ectopic tissue may display any disease affecting the thyroid, including malignancies, which have an estimated incidence of less than 1% [14].

Since 1910, only 52 cases of thyroid cancer arising from ectopic thyroid have been reported [61].

Toxic Adenoma

Toxic adenoma in children is rare and its estimated prevalence range from 0.7% to 5% of thyroid nodules [38, 63].

These nodules cause frequently compression symptoms due to the greater nodule size than in euthyroid patients [38].

In toxic adenoma, histology is almost always benign [4].

Differential Diagnosis

The differential diagnosis of thyroid nodules in children should include benign thyroid conditions such as [5]:

- Congenital hypothyroidism due to dyshormonogenesis or ectopy
- thyroid hemiagenesis
- thyroglossal duct cyst
- simple goiter
- cystic lesion
- nodular hyperplasia
- follicular adenoma
- Graves' disease and Hashimoto thyroiditis, all of which can predispose to the development of thyroid nodules.

Classification

The AJCC TNM Classification System should be used to describe the extent of disease in pediatric patients with differentiated thyroid cancer [64].

In the TNM classification all patients under 45 years have either stage I (no distant metastases) or stage II disease (with distant metastases)

Treatment

Goal

The goals of primary treatment of juvenile carcinoma are to eradicate disease and extend not only overall, but also recurrence-free survival.

For the other presentations, the aim of treatment depends of the pathology.

Means

Surgical Therapy

Preoperative Assessment

A complete head and neck physical examination is necessary for all thyroid nodules. This examination must include an assessment of the vocal cord function by nasofibroscopy that is better tolerated than indirect mirror laryngoscopy.

Neck USG to explore the thyroid gland and all regions of the neck in order to optimize the pre-operative surgical plan. Cytological confirmation of metastatic disease to lymph nodes in the lateral neck is recommended prior to surgery (ATA recommendation) [51].

Morphological exploration (MRI or CT) are not systematically performed and should explore patients with large or fixed thyroid masses, vocal cord paralysis, or bulky metastatic lymphadenopathy [65].

Nerve Monitoring

The use of intra-operative recurrent laryngeal nerve monitoring may be considered as an adjunct monitoring device, and may be considered for younger patients (<10 years of age), in patients undergoing central neck dissection, and in patients undergoing repeat surgical procedures [12].

Surgical Intervention

Thyroid Surgery

Different surgical options are performed for the management of thyroid diseases including [51]:

- Lobectomy
- Near total thyroidectomy
- Total thyroidectomy.

In our practice, we perform only lobectomy or total thyroidectomy.

The recurrent laryngeal nerve must be meticulously dissected and preserved to decrease the risk of permanent damage. The parathyroid glands are preserved and not over dissected to preserve their vascularization.

Cervical Lymphadenectomy

- The central neck dissection could be prophylactic (clinically/ radiographically node positive) or therapeutic (clinically/ radiographically node negative), ipsilateral or bilateral [66]
- Therapeutic lateral neck dissection include: levels III, IV, anterior V, and II [51]
- Because of the rarity of lymph node metastases superior to the spinal accessory nerve, some teams avoid routine dissection of levels IIB and

VA when there are no clinically or radiographically evident lymph node metastases [67].

Postoperative Management

- The main surgical complications after thyroidectomy are hypoparathyroidism and recurrent laryngeal nerve injury.
- There is an increased risk of complications in patients younger than 10 years of age, lymph node dissection, and repeat or extensive surgery [51].
- Many studies confirmed the notion that children with thyroid carcinoma have lower rates of complications when surgery is performed by experienced thyroid surgeons [14, 51]. Thus, all surgical procedures should be performed by high-volume, experienced endocrine, pediatric, and head and neck surgeons [68].
- Hypocalcemia (secondary to hypoparathyroidism), can be transient or permanent is the most common complication after thyroidectomy with an average rate of 5-15% [51]. Monitoring of calcium levels is performed every 4 to 8 hours until stability is reached [14]. Postoperative iPTH measurement can help to predict which patients would benefit from more intensive monitoring and treatment [51].
- Recurrent laryngeal nerve paralysis (temporary or permanent) either unilateral or bilateral is not rare. During surgery, careful dissection of the nerve, nerve monitoring (if available), and the choice of hemostatic techniques are important to prevent nerve palsy.

Radioactive Iodine Therapy (RAI)

The RAI in pediatric age should be preferably administered in capsule form, in association with an antiemetic medication, in an attempt to ensure that the activity administered has been fully ingested [12].

RAI is used in cases of follicular or papillary cancer for the purpose of both surveillance for occult metastatic or residual disease (^{123}I) and ablation of this residual disease (^{131}I) [69].

If ^{131}I is prescribed, the TSH should be above 30 mIU/L to facilitate uptake. The majority of children will achieve this level of TSH by $\geq$ 14 days of LT4 withdrawal [70, 51].

Use of recombinant human TSH (rhTSH) as a radioiodine therapy preparation method spares patients symptomatic hypothyroidism and its drawbacks, and may decrease radiation burden to healthy tissues [70].

For remnant ablation in adults, most centers use 3.7GBq (100 mCi) or 1.1GBq (30 mCi), which has been suggested to be the lowest effective activity in this setting, while others choose intermediate activities like 2.2GBq (60 mCi) [70]. This protocol is revised for children by giving 3.7 MBq/kg (1 mCi/kg) of body weight (range 1.85–7.4 MBq/kg, equal to 0.5–2 mCi/kg) [71].

The ATA recommend a posttreatment whole body scan for all children 4-7 days after 131I therapy [51].

Complications of RAI

There are both acute and long-term side effects and complications associated with exposure to therapeutic 131I [72]:

- temporary loss of salivary flow and change of taste (up to 30% of the cases)
- permanent xerostomia is rare
- leukemia
- pulmonary fibrosis that may occur in up to 1% (> 600 mci)
- transitional impairment of spermatogenesis and permanent sterility
- reversible menstrual changes and even infertility and early menopause

Thyroid Hormone Suppression Therapy

- Levothyroxine (LT4) suppression therapy has been prescribed to reduce nodule size or to reduce the risk of subsequent nodule formation [51].

A study of 78 children with benign thyroid nodules reported more than 50% reduction in nodule size in 30.6% of the group receiving a mean dose of levothyroxine of 1.69 μg/kg/day, while both palpable nodules and symptoms increased the non-treatment group [73].

- Thyroid hormone therapy with high doses of LT4 given for differentiated thyroid cancer suppress serum TSH to subnormal levels can limit both normal and malignant cell proliferation and, therefore, plays a significant role in the prevention of progression and recurrence [70].

Indications

Benign Nodule on FNA

Lesions reported as benign on FNA should undergo clinical follow-up [4].

These lesions should be followed by serial USG and undergo repeat FNA if suspicious features develop or the lesion continues to grow [51].

The 2015 ATA pediatric guidelines indicate that surgery (lobectomy or isthmusectomy) is favored over repeat FNA for most nodules with indeterminate cytology due to the apparent increased probability of malignancy among these indeterminate categories in children [51].

Indication of surgery in selected patients with benign nodule on FNA are [51, 2]:

- compressive symptoms
- cosmetic concerns
- patient or parent preference
- apparently benign solid thyroid nodules > 4cm
- lesions demonstrating significant growth (defined in adults as a ≥50% increase in volume or ≥20% increase in at least two dimensions)
- other clinical concerns for malignancy.

Toxic Adenoma

Surgical resection is the usual recommendation for toxic adenoma in children and adolescents [51, 4].

Differentiated Thyroid Cancer (DTC)

Due to the increased incidence of bilateral and multifocal disease in papillary carcinoma, total thyroidectomy is recommended in pediatric patients [74, 35, 51]. After total thyroidectomy, thyroid remnant volume should be less than 2 g on USG performed no earlier than 1 month after the procedure [75].

Complete thyroid resection allows for more efficacious therapy with RAI and allows for surveillance with serum thyroglobulin levels.

In Children with malignant cytology and clinical evidence of extrathyroidal invasion and/or loco-regional metastasis on pre-operative staging or intra-operative findings, a therapeutic central neck dissection (CND) should be performed [51]. In patients with unifocal disease, data from adult patients suggests that ipsilateral, prophylactic CND may provide the same potential benefit while decreasing the higher complication rate associated with bilateral CND [51, 76].

The USG appearance of the lymph nodes or at best confirmed metastasis to the lateral neck lymph nodes by FNA allow to pursue lateral lymph node dissection. Whereas routine prophylactic lateral neck dissection (levels III, IV, anterior V, and II) is not recommended [51].

In a study of 235 patients diagnosed with DTC before age 18, Handkiewicz-Junak et al. demonstrated that extensive initial therapy, consisting of total thyroidectomy combined with modified lymphadenectomy performed in cases of lymph node metastases and followed by radioiodine therapy was associated with a substantial decrease of locoregional recurrence risk. Postoperative staging performed within 12 weeks after surgery to evaluate who may or may not benefit from further therapy, to include additional surgery or ^{131}I therapy [51]. The ATA include Children with DTC into 3 risk levels (Table 4) [51].

Table 4. ATA Pediatric Thyroid Cancer Risk Levels [51]

ATA Risk Level	Definition
ATA PediatricLow-Risk	Disease grossly confined to the thyroid with N0/Nx disease or patients with incidental N1a disease (microscopic metastasis to a small number of central neck lymph nodes)
ATA Pediatric Intermediate Risk	Extensive N1a or minimal N1b disease
ATA Pediatric High-Risk	Regionally extensive disease (extensive N1b) or locally invasive disease (T4 tumors), with or without distant metastasis

In the AJCC TNM classification system:
N1a:Metastasis to Level VI
N1b: Metastasis to unilateral, bilateral, or contralateral cervical Levels I, II, III,IV, or V or retropharyngeal or Level VII
T4: Tumor extends beyond the thyroid capsule to invade subcutaneous soft tissues, larynx, trachea, esophagus, or recurrent laryngeal nerve (T4a) and Tumor invades prevertebral fascia or encases carotid artery or mediastinal vessels (T4b)

Due to its superior imaging quality and lower absorbed doses of radiation to the tissues, ^{123}I is used for the diagnostic whole body scan [69] [51]. After the initial staging, the follow up depend on the ATA risk levels [51]:

- ATA Pediatric Low Risk patients: initially assessed and followed with a TSH-suppressed Tg alone.
- ATA Pediatric Intermediate- and High-Risk patients: a TSH-stimulated Tg and a diagnostic whole body scan (DxWBS) is typically recommended to assess for evidence of persistent disease.

Neck US and/or hybrid imaging using SPECT/CT, may be used conjunctively to more accurately define the anatomic location of RAI uptake noted on a DxWBS [51]. PET/CT performed using 370MBq [18] F-FDG and standard CT can improve the diagnostic accuracy in patients with metastatic thyroid cancer, especially those that are iodine-negative DTC [77].

Once the diagnostic the initial staging is performed, ^{131}I is indicated for treatment of iodine-avid persistent locoregional or nodal disease that cannot be resected or presumed iodine-avid distant metastases [70]. However, routine ^{131}I therapy is advocated by some authors for children with T3 tumors (> 4 cm, limited to the thyroid, or any tumor with minimal extrathyroid extension) or extensive regional nodal involvement [70]. TSH suppression in children with DTC should be determined by ATA Pediatric Risk level:

- TSH Goal in ATA Pediatric Low-Risk = 0.5 – 1.0 mIU/L
- TSH Goal in ATA Pediatric Intermediate-Risk= 0.1 – 0.5 mIU/L
- TSH Goal in ATA Pediatric High-Risk < 0.1 mIU/L

Persistent or Recurrent Cervical Disease

- Patients with cervical RAI uptake due to disease that is small (<1 cm) or that cannot be visualized via imaging can be considered for therapeutic ^{131}I [70, 51].
- Patients with structural disease greater than 1 cm in size that is visualized by US and/or anatomic imaging (CT or MRI) and confirmed via FNA, surgical resection is preferable to ^{131}I. Thus, a high-volume thyroid surgeon should assess these patients [78].

Pulmonary Metastases

- Pediatric metastatic DTC appears to be more radioiodine-sensitive than adult disease, resulting in better survival in children [14].
- Children with RAI-avid pulmonary metastases visualized with a DxWBS are good candidates for ^{131}I therapy [51].

Incidental Papillary Thyroid Cancer Identified After Surgery

- Small foci of PTC may be incidentally discovered on histological examination of thyroid tissue resected for other benign diseases
- Neck USG is recommended to detect contralateral disease or disease in the regional lymph nodes.
- Completion thyroidectomy is required in those children who had less than a total thyroidectomy if there is USG evidence and cytologic confirmation of contralateral thyroid disease or malignant lymphadenopathy [51].

Follicular Thyroid Cancer (FTC)

- Patients with clear evidence of vascular invasion (> 3 involved blood vessels), known distant metastasis, and/or tumor size > 4 cm ➔ total thyroidectomy and staged postoperatively with RAI.
- Minimally-invasive FTC < 4 cm in size and with no or minimal vascular invasion (≤ 3 involved blood vessels) should be treated on a case-by-case basis but lobectomy alone may be sufficient.

Medullary Thyroid Carcinoma (MTC)

Total thyroidectomy and prophylactic central lymph node dissection make the mainstay for the treatment of MTC in both adults and children [36].

Advances in our understanding of the genotype–phenotype relationship have allowed for the development of guidelines to direct the timing of prophylactic total thyroidectomy, depending on patient-specific RET mutations [68].

In 2009, American Thyroid Association (ATA) issued evidence-based guidelines regarding the management of MTC. Mutations are classified based on time to development of MTC and stratified from A to D (Table 5):

- Risk D mutations (with mutation at codon 918) require prophylactic thyroidectomy within the first year of life
- The ATA suggests surgery before age five for A, B, and C mutations, with specific clinical criteria for exception [68, 79].

Table 5. American Thyroid Association (ATA) risk level and prophylactic thyroidectomy testing and therapy [68]

ATA risk level	*Age of RET testing*	*Age of required first US*	*Age of required first serum Ct*	*Age of prophylactic surgery*
D	ASAP and within the 1st year of life	ASAP and within the 1st year of life	6 months, if surgery not already done	ASAP and within the 1st year of life
C	<3–5 years	>3–5 years	>3–5 years	Before age 5 years
B	<3–5 years	>3–5 years	>3–5 years	Consider surgery before age 5. May delay surgery beyond age 5 years if stringent criteria are met.[a]
A	<3–5 years	>3–5 years	>3–5 years	May delay surgery beyond age 5 years if stringent criteria are met.[a]

a: A normal annual basal stimulated* serum Ct, normal annual neck US, less aggressive MTC family history, and family preference.
ASAP, as soon as possible

In patients with hereditary or sporadic MTC diagnosed clinically, the ATA guidelines suggest total thyroidectomy and central neck dissection, along with lateral compartment lymph node dissection for clinically or radiographically evident lymphadenopthy [79].

Replacement rather than suppressive T 4 therapy with target serum TSH levels between 0.5 and 2.5 mIU/L is recommended for patients with MTC [79].

Follow-Up

Differentiated Thyroid Cancer

Patients are typically seen at 1 month, 3 months, 6 months, and 1 year following surgery, after which they are followed annually.

We propose the ATA follow-up method:

- TSH for adaptation of thyroid hormone suppression therapy.
- Tg serves as a sensitive tumor marker in the evaluation, treatment, and long-term follow up of DTC in children, even in children not previously treated with RAI. Serum anti-thyroglobulin antibodies (TgAb) levels should be simultaneously measured in all samples as the presence of TgAb will render the Tg result uninterpretable [51].
- Neck USG should be performed at least 6 months after initial surgery and then at 6-12 month intervals for ATA Pediatric Intermediate- and High-Risk patients and at annual intervals for ATA Pediatric Low-Risk patients. Follow-up beyond 5 years should be individualized based on recurrence risk [51].
- A DxWBS should be performed after at least 12 months of clinical follow-up in children with ATA Pediatric High-Risk disease who were previously treated with ^{131}I or known to have iodine-avid metastatic disease based upon a previous posttreatment scan [51].

Medullary Carcinoma

Serum calcitonin should be measured 2–3 months postoperatively for early detection of recurrence [79]. Postoperative MTC patients with detectable serum calcitonin levels <150 pg/mL should be evaluated with neck US [79].

In addition to neck US, postoperative MTC patients with serum Ct levels >150 pg/mL should undergo additional imaging techniques to evaluate for distant metastases [79].

Outcomes

Despite having a greater recurrence rate, when compared to adults, survival seems to be better in pediatric patients [80].

In a large cohort of 740 pediatric patients with thyroid cancer, the 5- and 10-year survival for the entire group was 99.5% and 98.8%, respectively [80].

In The Surveillance, Epidemiology, and End Results (SEER) registry from 1973 to 2004, Hogan et al. studied the outcomes of 1753 patients with thyroid carcinoma less than 20 y of age and found that the overall mean survival time was 30.5 years. In the same study, patients with medullary cancer had significantly shorter mean survival than those with papillary cancer [31].

The 5-year survival of sporadic and hereditary MTC ranges from 70% to 90% and 10-year survival from 56% to 87% [81].

Prognosis

The greater risk for more extensive disease or higher rates of recurrence is associated with [80] younger children (<10-15 years of age), presence of residual cervical disease, children operated on using a less extensive approach than total thyroidectomy.

In the largest study including 740 children from Belarus independent parameters significantly associated with the risk of recurrent nodal disease were [80]:

- young age at diagnosis
- multifocal carcinomas
- N1 status
- lack of neck lymph node dissection.

In the same study [80], the significant risk factors for lung metastases were female gender, young age at diagnosis, and the presence of symptoms.

Hogan et al. [31] found that male gender, nonpapillary histology, distant disease, and no surgery were all independent prognostic factors of the worse outcome. For patients with medullary thyroid carcinoma, radiation therapy was also identified as an independent predictor of lower survival [31].

Conclusion

The incidence of clinically palpable thyroid nodules in children is estimated to be around 1–2%.

When compared to adults, pediatric thyroid nodules behave differently, as the rate of malignancy in pediatric nodules may be as high as 25% compared with the rate of 5% in adult nodules.

The current treatment recommendation of pediatric thyroid cancer is total thyroidectomy and central lymphadenectomy, with modified lateral lymphadenectomy in case of biopsy-proven metastases, and followed by radioiodine ablation for the differentiated carcinomas.

In these young patients, surgery should be performed by an experienced thyroid surgeon at a tertiary care pediatric medical center should perform surgery. Despite having a greater recurrence rate, when compared to adults, prognosis seems to be better in pediatric patients.

References

[1] Izquierdo R, Shankar R, Kort K, Khurana K. Ultrasound-guided fine-needle aspiration in the management of thyroid nodules in children and adolescents. *Thyroid.* 2009 Jul;19(7):703-5.

[2] Guille JT, Opoku-Boateng A, Thibeault SL, Chen H. Evaluation and management of the pediatric thyroid nodule. *Oncologist.* 2015 Jan;20(1):19-27.

[3] Scholz S, Smith JR, Chaignaud B, Shamberger RC, Huang SA. Thyroid surgery at Children's Hospital Boston: a 35-year single-institution experience. *J Pediatr Surg*. 2011 Mar;46(3):437-42.

[4] Corrias A, Mussa A. Thyroid nodules in pediatrics: which ones can be left alone, which ones must be investigated, when and how. *J Clin Res Pediatr Endocrinol*. 2013;5 Suppl 1:57-69.

[5] Niedziela M. Pathogenesis, diagnosis and management of thyroid nodules in children. *Endocr Relat Cancer*. 2006 Jun;13(2):427-53.

[6] Grigsby PW, Gal-or A, Michalski JM, Doherty GM. Childhood and adolescent thyroid carcinoma. *Cancer*. 2002 Aug 15;95(4):724-9.

[7] Wood JH, Partrick DA, Barham HP, Bensard DD, Travers SH, Bruny JL, McIntyre RC Jr. Pediatric thyroidectomy: a collaborative surgical approach. *J Pediatr Surg*. 2011 May;46(5):823-8. .

[8] Dean DS, Gharib H. Epidemiology of thyroid nodules. *Best Pract Res Clin Endocrinol Metab*. 2008 Dec;22(6):901-11.

[9] Gharib H, Papini E. Thyroid nodules: clinical importance, assessment, and treatment. *Endocrinol Metab Clin North Am*. 2007 Sep;36(3):707-35, vi.

[10] Rallison ML, Dobyns BM, Meikle AW, Bishop M, Lyon JL, Stevens W. Natural history of thyroid abnormalities: prevalence, incidence, and regression of thyroid diseases in adolescents and young adults. *Am J Med.* 1991 Oct;91(4):363-70.

[11] Trowbridge FL, Matovinovic J, McLaren GD, Nichaman MZ. Iodine and goiter in children. *Pediatrics*. 1975 Jul;56(1):82-90.

[12] Vaisman F, Corbo R, Vaisman M. Thyroid carcinoma in children and adolescents-systematic review of the literature. *J Thyroid Res.* 2011;2011:845362.

[13] Safford SD, Skinner MA. Thyroid and parathyroid disease in children. *Semin Pediatr Surg*. 2006 May;15(2):85-91.

[14] Jatana KR, Zimmerman D. Pediatric thyroid nodules and malignancy. *Otolaryngol Clin North Am*. 2015 Feb;48(1):47-58.

[15] Rahbar, Reza. Pediatric head and neck tumors: A-Z guide to presentation and multimodality management. Springer,New York (US) , 2014; pp 369-378.

[16] Sigurdson AJ, Ronckers CM, Mertens AC, Stovall M, Smith SA, Liu Y, Berkow RL, Hammond S, Neglia JP, Meadows AT, Sklar CA, Robison LL, Inskip PD. Primary thyroid cancer after a first tumour in childhood (the Childhood Cancer Survivor Study): a nested case-control study. *Lancet.* 2005 Jun 11-17;365(9476):2014-23.

[17] Ron E, Lubin JH, Shore RE, Mabuchi K, Modan B, Pottern LM, Schneider AB, Tucker MA, Boice JD Jr. Thyroid cancer after exposure to external radiation: a pooled analysis of seven studies. *Radiat Res.* 1995 Mar;141(3):259-77.

[18] Catelinois O, Verger P, Colonna M, Rogel A, Hemon D, Tirmarche M. Projecting the time trend of thyroid cancers: its impact on assessment of radiation-induced cancer risks. *Health Phys*. 2004 Dec;87(6):606-14.

[19] Shore RE. Issues and epidemiological evidence regarding radiation-induced thyroid cancer. *Radiat Res.* 1992 Jul;131(1):98-111.

[20] Shibata Y, Yamashita S, Masyakin VB, Panasyuk GD, Nagataki S. 15 years after Chernobyl: new evidence of thyroid cancer. *Lancet.* 2001 Dec 8;358(9297):1965-6.

[21] Mahoney MC, Lawvere S, Falkner KL, Averkin YI, Ostapenko VA, Michalek AM, Moysich KB, McCarthy PL. Thyroid cancer incidence trends in Belarus: examining the impact of Chernobyl. *Int J Epidemiol.* 2004 Oct;33(5):1025-33.

[22] Cohen A, Rovelli A, Merlo DF, van Lint MT, Lanino E, Bresters D, Ceppi M, Bocchini V, Tichelli A, Socié G. Risk for secondary thyroid carcinoma after hematopoietic stem-cell transplantation: an EBMT Late Effects Working Party Study. *J Clin Oncol.* 2007 Jun 10;25(17):2449-54.

[23] Smith MB, Xue H, Strong L, Takahashi H, Jaffe N, Ried H, Zietz H, Andrassy RJ. Forty-year experience with second malignancies after treatment of childhood cancer: analysis of outcome following the

development of the second malignancy. *J Pediatr Surg.* 1993 Oct;28(10):1342-8; discussion 1348-9.

[24] Yip FW, Reeve TS, Poole AG, Delbridge L. Thyroid nodules in childhood and adolescence. Aust N Z J Surg. 1994 Oct;64(10):676-8.

[25] Gingalewski CA, Newman KD. Seminars: controversies in the management of pediatric thyroid malignancy. *J Surg Oncol.* 2006 Dec 15;94(8):748-52.

[26] Gandhi M, Evdokimova V, Nikiforov YE. Mechanisms of chromosomal rearrangements in solid tumors: the model of papillary thyroid carcinoma. *Mol Cell Endocrinol.* 2010 May 28;321(1):36-43.

[27] Bongarzone I, Butti MG, Coronelli S, Borrello MG, Santoro M, Mondellini P, Pilotti S, Fusco A, Della Porta G, Pierotti MA. Frequent activation of ret protooncogene by fusion with a new activating gene in papillary thyroid carcinomas. *Cancer Res.* 1994 Jun 1;54(11):2979-85.

[28] Bongarzone I, Fugazzola L, Vigneri P, Mariani L, Mondellini P, Pacini F, Basolo F, Pinchera A, Pilotti S, Pierotti MA. Age-related activation of the tyrosine kinase receptor protooncogenes RET and NTRK1 in papillary thyroid carcinoma. *J Clin Endocrinol Metab.* 1996 May;81(5):2006-9.

[29] Yamashita S, Saenko V. Mechanisms of Disease: molecular genetics of childhood thyroid cancers. *Nat Clin Pract Endocrinol Metab.* 2007 May;3(5):422-9.

[30] DeLellis RA, Lloyd RV, Heitz PU, Eng C 2004 Pathology and Genetics of Tumours of. Pathology and Genetics of Tumours of Endocrine Organs World Health Organization Classification of Tumours, Volume 8. IARC Press, Lyon, France.

[31] Hogan AR, Zhuge Y, Perez EA, Koniaris LG, Lew JI, Sola JE. Pediatric thyroid carcinoma: incidence and outcomes in 1753 patients. *J Surg Res.* 2009 Sep;156(1):167-72.

[32] Steliarova-Foucher E, Stiller CA, Pukkala E, Lacour B, Plesko I, Parkin DM. Thyroid cancer incidence and survival among European children and adolescents (1978-1997): report from the Automated Childhood Cancer Information System project. *Eur J Cancer.* 2006 Sep;42(13):2150-69.

[33] Roy R, Kouniavsky G, Schneider E, Allendorf JD, Chabot JA, Logerfo P, Dackiw AP, Colombani P, Zeiger MA, Lee JA. Predictive factors of malignancy in pediatric thyroid nodules. *Surgery.* 2011 Dec;150(6):1228-33.

[34] Osipoff JN, Wilson TA. Consultation with the specialist: thyroid nodules. *Pediatr Rev.* 2012 Feb;33(2):75-81; quiz 82. doi: 10.1542/pir.33-2-75.

[35] Önder A, Aycan Z. Approach to thyroid nodules in children and adolescents. *Turk J Pediatr.* 2014 May-Jun;56(3):219-25.

[36] Viola D, Romei C, Elisei R. Medullary thyroid carcinoma in children. *Endocr Dev.* 2014;26:202-13.

[37] Cooper DS, Doherty GM, Haugen BR, Kloos RT, Lee SL, Mandel SJ, Mazzaferri EL, McIver B, Sherman SI, Tuttle RM et Taskforce., American Thyroid Association Guidelines. Management guidelines for patients with thyroid nodules and differentiated thyroid cancer. *Thyroid.* 2006 Feb;16(2):109-42.

[38] Corrias A, Mussa A, Baronio F, Arrigo T, Salerno M, Segni M, Vigone MC, Gastaldi R, Zirilli G, Tuli G, Beccaria L, Iughetti L, Einaudi S, Weber G, De Luca F, Cassio A et Di, Study Group for Thyroid Diseases of Italian Society for Pediatric Endocrinology and. Diagnostic features of thyroid nodules in pediatrics. *Arch Pediatr Adolesc Med.* 2010 Aug;164(8):714-9.

[39] Mussa A, Salerno MC, Bona G, Wasniewska M, Segni M, Cassio A, Vigone MC, Gastaldi R, Iughetti L, Santanera A, Capalbo D, Matarazzo P, De Luca F, Weber G, Corrias A. Serum thyrotropin concentration in children with isolated thyroid nodules. *J Pediatr.* 2013 Nov;163(5):1465-70.

[40] Pacini F, Schlumberger M, Dralle H, Elisei R, Smit JW, Wiersinga W et Taskforce., European Thyroid Cancer. European consensus for the management of patients with differentiated thyroid carcinoma of the follicular epithelium. *Eur J Endocrinol.* 2006 Jun;154(6):787-803.

[41] Wells SA Jr, Asa SL, Dralle H, Elisei R, Evans DB, Gagel RF, Lee N, Machens A, Moley JF, Pacini F, Raue F, Frank-Raue K, Robinson B, Rosenthal MS, Santoro M, Schlumberger M, Shah M, Waguespack SG. Revised american thyroid association guidelines for the management of medullary thyroid carcinoma. *Thyroid.* 2015 Jun;25(6):567-610.

[42] Guarino E, Tarantini B, Pilli T, Checchi S, Brilli L, Ciuoli C, Di Cairano G, Mazzucato P, Pacini F. Presurgical serum thyroglobulin has no prognostic value in papillary thyroid cancer. *Thyroid.* 2005 Sep;15(9):1041-5.

[43] Grani G, Fumarola A. Thyroglobulin in lymph node fine-needle aspiration washout: a systematic review and meta-analysis of diagnostic accuracy. *J Clin Endocrinol Metab.* 2014 Jun;99(6):1970-82.

[44] De Crea C, Raffaelli M, Maccora D, Carrozza C, Canu G, Fadda G, Bellantone R, Lombardi CP. Calcitonin measurement in fine-needle aspirate washouts vs. cytologic examination for diagnosis of primary or metastatic medullary thyroid carcinoma. *Acta Otorhinolaryngol Ital.* 2014 Dec;34(6):399-405.

[45] Goldfarb M, Gondek SS, Sanchez Y, Lew JI. Clinic-based ultrasound can predict malignancy in pediatric thyroid nodules. *Thyroid.* 2012 Aug;22(8):827-31.

[46] Sun J, Cai J, Wang X. Real-time ultrasound elastography for differentiation of benign and malignant thyroid nodules: a meta-analysis. *J Ultrasound Med.* 2014 Mar;33(3):495-502.

[47] McHenry CR, Danish R, Murphy T, Marty JJ. Atypical thyroglossal duct cyst: a rare cause for a solitary cold thyroid nodule in childhood. *Am Surg.* 1993 Apr;59(4):223-8.

[48] Mazzaferri EL. Management of a solitary thyroid nodule. *N Engl J Med.* 1993 Feb 25;328(8):553-9.

[49] Papendieck P, Gruñeiro-Papendieck L, Venara M, Acha O, Cozzani H, Mateos F, Maglio S, Calcagno ML, Bergada I, Chiesa A. Differentiated Thyroid Cancer in Children: Prevalence and Predictors in a Large Cohort with Thyroid Nodules Followed Prospectively. *J Pediatr.* 2015 Jul;167(1):199-201.

[50] Izquierdo R, Arekat MR, Knudson PE, Kartun KF, Khurana K, Kort K, Numann PJ. Comparison of palpation-guided versus ultrasound-guided fine-needle aspiration biopsies of thyroid nodules in an outpatient endocrinology practice. *Endocr Pract.* 2006 Nov-Dec;12(6):609-14.

[51] Francis GL, Waguespack SG, Bauer AJ, Angelos P, Benvenga S, Cerutti JM, Dinauer CA, Hamilton J, Hay ID, Luster M, Parisi MT, Rachmiel M, Thompson GB, Yamashita S. Management Guidelines for Children with Thyroid Nodules and Differentiated Thyroid Cancer. *Thyroid.* 2015 Jul;25(7):716-59. doi: 10.1089/thy.2014.0460.

[52] Cibas ES. Fine-needle aspiration in the work-up of thyroid nodules. Otolaryngol Clin North Am. 2010 Apr;43(2):257-71, vii-viii. doi: 10.1016/j.otc.2010.01.003.

[53] Norlén O, Charlton A, Sarkis LM, Henwood T, Shun A, Gill AJ, Delbridge L. Risk of malignancy for each Bethesda class in pediatric thyroid nodules. *J Pediatr Surg.* 2015 Jul;50(7):1147-9.

[54] Smith M, Pantanowitz L, Khalbuss WE, Benkovich VA, Monaco SE. Indeterminate pediatric thyroid fine needle aspirations: a study of 68 cases. *Acta Cytol.* 2013;57(4):341-8. .

[55] Kouniavsky G, Zeiger MA. The quest for diagnostic molecular markers for thyroid nodules with indeterminate or suspicious cytology. *J Surg Oncol.* 2012 Apr 1;105(5):438-43.

[56] Keutgen XM1, Filicori F, Fahey TJ 3rd. Molecular diagnosis for indeterminate thyroid nodules on fine needle aspiration: advances and limitations. *Expert Rev Mol Diagn.* 2013 Jul;13(6):613-23.

[57] Corrias A, Einaudi S, Chiorboli E, Weber G, Crino A, Andreo M, Cesaretti G, Sanctis L, de, Messina MF, Segni M, Cicchetti M, Vigone M, Pasquino AM, Spera S, Luca F, de, Mussa GC, Bona G. Accuracy of fine needle aspiration biopsy of thyroid nodules in detecting malignancy in childhood: comparison with conventional clinical, laboratory, and imaging approaches. . *J Clin Endocrinol Metab.* 2001;86:4644–4648.

[58] Forest VI, Murali R, Clark JR. Thyroglossal duct cyst carcinoma: case series. *J Otolaryngol Head Neck Surg.* 2011 Apr;40(2):151-6.

[59] Pfeiffer MS, Kim GH, Krishnan M. Thyroglossal duct papillary carcinoma in a 15-year old female and review of pediatric cases of thyroglossal duct carcinoma. *Int J Pediatr Otorhinolaryngol.* 2014 Jan;78(1):135-8.

[60] Noussios G, Anagnostis P, Goulis DG, Lappas D, Natsis K. Ectopic thyroid tissue: anatomical, clinical, and surgical implications of a rare entity. *Eur J Endocrinol.* 2011 Sep;165(3):375-82.

[61] 61.Sturniolo G1, Violi MA, Galletti B, Baldari S, Campennì A, Vermiglio F, Moleti M. Differentiated thyroid carcinoma in lingual thyroid. *Endocrine.* 2015 May 19 [Epub ahead of. print]

[62] Guerra G, Cinelli M, Mesolella M, Tafuri D, Rocca A, Amato B, Rengo S, Testa D. Morphological, diagnostic and surgical features of ectopic thyroid gland: a review of literature. *Int J Surg.* 2014;12 Suppl 1:S3-11.

[63] Tonacchera M, Pinchera A, Vitti P. Assessment of nodular goitre. *Best Pract Res Clin Endocrinol Metab.* 2010 Feb;24(1):51-61.

[64] International Union Against Cancer (UICC). TNM Classification of Malignant Tumors, Wiley, New York, NY, USA, 7th edition, 2009.

[65] Choi JS, Kim J, Kwak JY, Kim MJ, Chang HS, Kim EK. Preoperative staging of papillary thyroid carcinoma: comparison of ultrasound imaging and CT. Choi JS1, Kim J, Kwak JY, Kim MJ, Chang HS, Kim EK. *AJR Am J Roentgenol.* 2009 Sep;193(3):871-8.

[66] Orloff LA, Kuppersmith RB. American Thyroid Association's central neck dissection terminology and classification for thyroid cancer consensus statement. *Otolaryngol Head Neck Surg.* 2010 Jan;142(1):4-5.

[67] Welch K, McHenry CR. Selective lateral compartment neck dissection for thyroid cancer. *J Surg Res*. 2013 Sep;184(1):193-9.

[68] Breuer C, Tuggle C, Solomon D, Sosa JA. Pediatric thyroid disease: when is surgery necessary, and who should be operating on our children? *J Clin Res Pediatr Endocrinol*. 2013;5 Suppl 1:79-85.

[69] Cohen JB, Kalinyak JE, McDougall IR. Clinical implications of the differences between diagnostic 123I and post-therapy 131I scans. *Nucl Med Commun*. 2004 Feb;25(2):129-34.

[70] Jarzab B, Handkiewicz-Junak D, Wloch J. Juvenile differentiated thyroid carcinoma and the role of radioiodine in its treatment: a qualitative review. *Endocr Relat Cancer*. 2005 Dec;12(4):773-803.

[71] Hung W, Sarlis NJ. Current controversies in the management of pediatric patients with well-differentiated nonmedullary thyroid cancer: a review. *Thyroid*. 2002 Aug;12(8):683-702.

[72] Van Santen HM, Aronson DC, Vulsma T, Tummers RF, Geenen MM, de Vijlder JJ, van den Bos C. Frequent adverse events after treatment for childhood-onset differentiated thyroid carcinoma: a single institute experience. *Eur J Cancer*. 2004 Jul;40(11):1743-51.

[73] Corrias A, Mussa A, Wasniewska M, Segni M, Cassio A, Salerno M, Gastaldi R, Vigone MC, Bal M, Matarazzo P, Weber G, De Luca F. Levothyroxine treatment in pediatric benign thyroid nodules. *Horm Res Paediatr*. 2011;75(4):246-51.

[74] Handkiewicz-Junak D, Wloch J, Roskosz J, Krajewska J, Kropinska A, Pomorski L, Kukulska A, Prokurat A, Wygoda Z, Jarzab B. Total thyroidectomy and adjuvant radioiodine treatment independently decrease locoregional recurrence risk in childhood and adolescent differentiated thyroid cancer. *J Nucl Med*. 2007 Jun;48(6):879-88.

[75] Mazzaferri EL, Massoll N. Management of papillary and follicular (differentiated) thyroid cancer: new paradigms using recombinant human thyrotropin. *Endocr Relat Cancer*. 2002 Dec;9(4):227-47.

[76] Moo TA, Umunna B, Kato M, Butriago D, Kundel A, Lee JA, Zarnegar R, Fahey TJ 3rd. Ipsilateral versus bilateral central neck lymph node dissection in papillary thyroid carcinoma. *Ann Surg*. 2009 Sep;250(3):403-8.

[77] Palmedo H, Bucerius J, Joe A, Strunk H, Hortling N, Meyka S, Roedel R, Wolff M, Wardelmann E, Biersack HJ, Jaeger U. Integrated PET/CT in differentiated thyroid cancer: diagnostic accuracy and impact on patient management. *J Nucl Med*. 2006 Apr;47(4):616-24.

[78] Clayman GL, Shellenberger TD, Ginsberg LE, Edeiken BS, El-Naggar AK, Sellin RV, Waguespack SG, Roberts DB, Mishra A, Sherman SI. Approach and safety of comprehensive central compartment dissection in patients with recurrent papillary thyroid carcinoma. *Head Neck*. 2009 Sep;31(9):1152-63.

[79] American Thyroid Association Guidelines Task Force, Kloos RT, Eng C, Evans DB, Francis GL, Gagel RF, Gharib H, Moley JF, Pacini F, Ringel MD, Schlumberger M, Wells SA Jr. Medullary thyroid cancer: management guidelines of the American Thyroid Association. *Thyroid.* 2009 Jun;19(6):565-612.

[80] Demidchik YE, Demidchik EP, Reiners C, Biko J, Mine M, Saenko VA, Yamashita S. Comprehensive clinical assessment of 740 cases of surgically treated thyroid cancer in children of Belarus. *Ann Surg*. 2006 Apr;243(4):525-32.

[81] Hu MI, Ying AK, Jimenez C. Update on medullary thyroid cancer. *Endocrinol Metab Clin North Am*. 2014 Jun;43(2):423-42.

In: Thyroid Nodules
Editor: Marsha Vasquez
ISBN: 978-1-63483-592-3

Chapter II

Role of Clinic-Based Ultrasound in the Management of Thyroid Nodules

Punam P. Parikh, M.D. and John I. Lew*, M.D., F.A.C.S.
DeWitt Daughtry Family Department of Surgery,
Division of Surgical Endocrinology,
University of Miami Leonard M. Miller School of Medicine,
Miami, Florida

Abstract

Since the late 1960's, ultrasound (US) has become essential in the examination of the thyroid gland with the increased availability of high-frequency linear array transducers and computer-enhanced imaging capabilities in a clinic-based setting. As a non-invasive, rapid and easily

* Correspondence: John I. Lew, M.D., F.A.C.S. Associate Professor of Surgery. Chief of Endocrine Surgery. University of Miami Leonard M. Miller School of Medicine. Physician Leader, Thyroid and Other Endocrine Cancer Site Disease Group. University of Miami Sylvester Comprehensive Cancer Center. Director, Fellowship in Endocrine Surgery. The DeWitt Daughtry Family Department of Surgery. University of Miami and Jackson Memorial Hospitals. 1120 NW 14th Street, CRB-Room 410P (M-875). Miami, FL 33136. Phone: (305) 243-4211. Fax: (305) 243-4221. JLew@miami.edu

reproducible imaging study, US has a broadened utility beyond the simple confirmation of thyroid nodules and their size. Clinic-based US can image thyroid lesions and provide additional information in real time with greater clarity that otherwise might have been missed by history and physical examination. The routine use of diagnostic imaging has led to the incidental discovery of many non-palpable thyroid nodules, most of which require further evaluation and management. Specifically, US has become useful in the qualitative analysis and delineation of such thyroid nodules based on features for malignancy or benignity. Furthermore, examination of cervical lymph node basins for staging purposes and characterization of the contralateral thyroid lobe are also achievable with clinic-based US, which may influence the extent of the intended thyroid operation. Additionally, US-guided fine-needle aspiration can be crucial in the preoperative investigation of a thyroid nodule. It provides accurate cytologic sampling from thyroid nodules thereby minimizing inconclusive specimens. This chapter discusses the role and utility of clinic-based US in the evaluation and management of thyroid nodules.

Introduction

Since the late 1960's, ultrasound (US) has become essential in the examination of the thyroid gland with the increased availability of high-frequency linear array transducers and computer-enhanced imaging capabilities in a clinic-based setting. As a non-invasive, rapid and easily reproducible imaging study, US has a broadened utility beyond the simple confirmation of thyroid nodules and their size. US not only is useful in the qualitative characterization of thyroid nodules based on benign or malignant features, but on the basis of such classifications and the relative risk for thyroid malignancy, performance of US elastography, US-guided fine-needle aspiration (FNA), preoperative staging, lymph node mapping and the extent of surgery can be subsequently determined in addition to the postoperative surveillance for recurrent thyroid cancer (Table 1).

Clinic-based US has become an integral part of clinical practice, where it has demonstrated great benefit to patients being evaluated and treated for thyroid cancer. Overall, unlike the incidence of thyroid nodules, thyroid cancer is uncommon. On clinical examination up to 4-7% of the adult population have thyroid nodules [1]. In contrast, the annual incidence of thyroid cancer is 2 per 100,000 women and 1 per 100,000 men, and it accounts for only 1% of all malignancies [2]. The prevalence of thyroid nodules increases with age and women are more commonly affected than men [3]. Excluding underlying malignancy in a thyroid nodule is imperative in high-risk patients who have a family history of thyroid cancer and radiation exposure in addition to aforementioned factors such as age and gender [4].

Table 1. Indications for Clinic-Based Ultrasound in the Management of Thyroid Nodules

1. Thyroid nodule size
2. Thyroid nodule features for benignity versus malignancy
3. Staging: evaluation of cervical lymph node basins
4. Ultrasound-guided fine-needle aspiration
5. Surveillance of disease recurrence postoperatively

Thyroid US is used to evaluate index nodule size, location, characteristics, and the number and presence of additional thyroid nodules (e.g., contralateral lobe). Patients with multiple thyroid nodules also have the same risk for malignancy as those with solitary nodules, and it is recommended that all patients with a nodular thyroid gland undergo US evaluation [5, 6]. Although no single US feature carries a high sensitivity and positive predictive value for thyroid cancer, there is evidence to suggest that a number of US characteristics, when occurring together, are associated with a higher risk for malignancy [7, 8].

Ultrasound Characterstics of Thyroid Nodules

A variety of US characteristics are thought to differentiate benign from malignant thyroid nodules. These US features include echogenicity, internal echo pattern, margins, shape/dimension ratio, calcifications, acoustic phenomenon, compressibility, and vascularity [5, 9]. Whereas the well-defined and smooth margins of a thyroid nodule may signify benignity, irregular or ill-defined lesions suggest malignancy (Figure 1).

Although benign thyroid nodules are more likely to be entirely cystic in nature, many malignant lesions are solid and appear hypoechoic relative to adjacent thyroid tissue. Furthermore, thyroid nodules with a spongiform appearance comprised of >50% multiple microcystic components are most likely benign [10, 11].

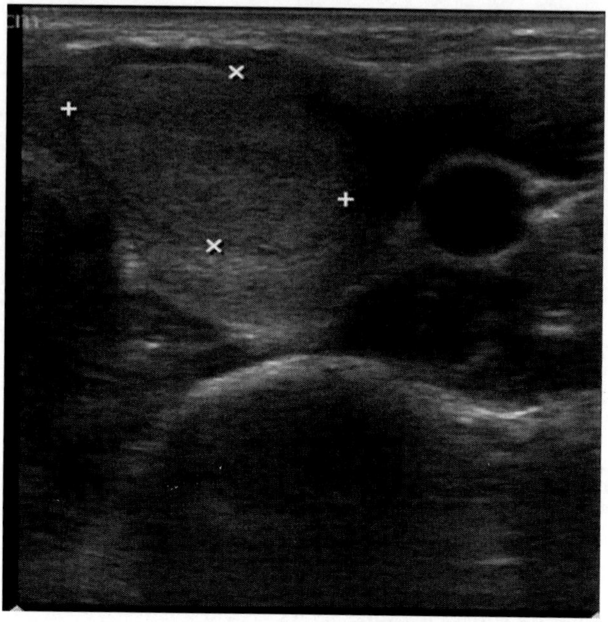

Figure 1. Ultrasound of benign thyroid nodule with well-defined and smooth margins.

A thyroid nodule defined as being greater in its anteroposterior than its transverse dimension (i.e., taller greater than wider) has been described as more likely to be malignant than benign (Figure 2) [9]. Thyroid nodules with microcalcifications are more strongly associated with malignancy than those with coarse or no calcifications (Figure 3). Central vascularity is more likely to be characteristic of malignant thyroid nodules, whereas peripheral vascularity is associated with benign lesions [5, 9]. Apart from the index nodule, the presence of suspicious-appearing lymph nodes is also associated with thyroid malignancy (Figure 4). Recent evidence suggests that the combination of hypoechogenicity, irregular borders, and microcalcifications in the same solitary thyroid nodule has the strongest correlation with differentiated thyroid cancer with a 30-fold higher risk for malignancy [8].

US elastography has been used for noninvasive differentiation between benign and malignant thyroid nodules in many studies [12-17], whereby significantly higher stiffness or less compressibility of thyroid nodules has been highly correlated with malignancy [12].

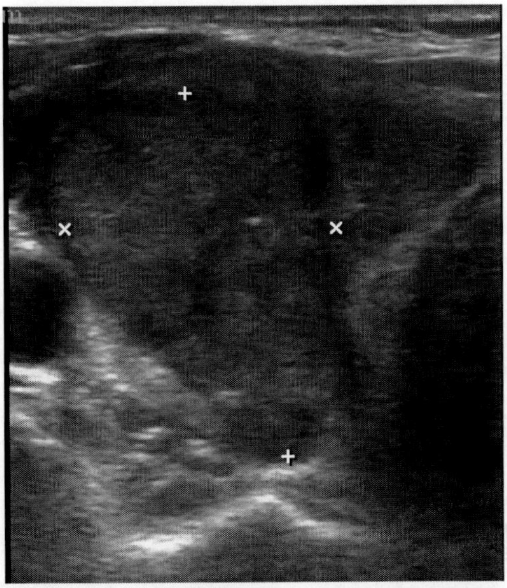

Figure 2. Taller greater than wider dimensions of thyroid nodule associated with malignancy.

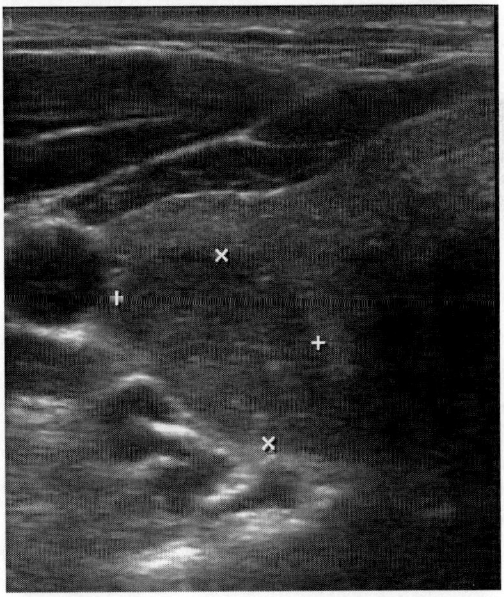

Figure 3. Ultrasound of malignant thyroid nodule with hypoechogenicity, ill-defined borders and microcalcifications.

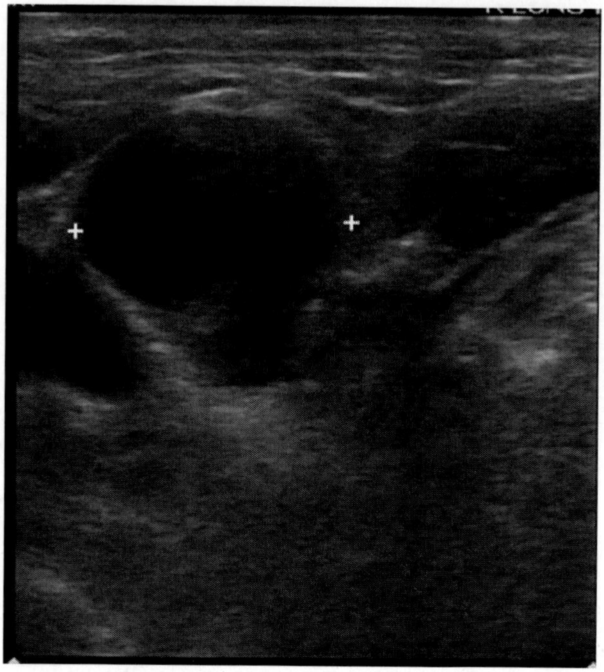

Figure 4. Ultrasound of malignant right level 2 lymph node.

Elastography measures the deformation of tissue in response to an applied force and derives and displays its stiffness, based on the fact that malignant nodules are stiffer than their benign counterparts [18]. Despite the high sensitivity and specificity values of up to 97% and 100% respectively reported in previous studies, a lack of inter-observer agreement has been identified as a major limitation of elastography using external compression [19, 20]. Lim et al. reported significant inter-observer and intra-observer agreement for US elastography using carotid artery pulsation rather than external compression [21, 22]. However, because US elastography imaging of the thyroid requires that the nodule be compressed (either externally or intrinsically) to derive its stiffness, performance can be influenced by several nodule parameters such as nodule location and size, which would affect the amount of intrinsic compression placed on the nodule.

A nodule's distance to the carotid artery can also significantly influence the diagnostic performance of US thyroid elastography during intrinsic compression [21]. The elasticity contrast index (ECI) quantifies the local strain contrast within a nodule [21]. For nodules within 10 mm of the carotid artery, especially when the probability of malignancy is high, caution should be used in the interpretation of elastography results [21]. When a nodule is very close to the carotid artery, a source of compression, its ECI value or the elasticity of the nodule tends to be low, especially in malignant nodules, as compared to malignant nodules located farther away from the carotid artery which manifest a higher ECI [21]. In general, however, a low ECI value is suggestive of benignity. However, a low ECI value in a nodule suspicious for malignancy located close to the carotid artery underestimates stiffness in the nodule and can lead to inaccurate diagnosis by elastography altogether [21].

Ultrasound Guided Fine Needle Aspiration of Thyroid Nodules

US allows for more selective FNA of thyroid nodules based on certain sonographic features and combination of features highly associated with malignancy [7, 23-25]. Whereas FNA has traditionally been routinely performed on palpable lesions, US-guided FNA can be performed more selectively in those patients with nonpalpable or subcentimeter thyroid nodules that have suspicious sonographic features, a previous history of thyroid cancer, a history of radiation exposure and a family history of thyroid cancer. US-guided FNA decreases the percentage of inadequate specimens while maintaining or increasing the sensitivity and specificity [26, 27]. The complementary use of US and FNA decreases the rate of false-negative results from needle misplacement and reduces the rate of nondiagnostic results. US-guided FNA in the clinic setting can be performed with a 91%–93% diagnostic accuracy rate, comparable with or better than those rates reported by radiologists and experienced cytopathologists [28, 29].

Ultrasound Staging of Thyroid Cancer

US has been used to preoperatively stage patients with well-differentiated thyroid cancer and to determine the extent of surgical resection, including formal neck dissection, in certain patients [25, 30]. The presence of >25% contact between papillary thyroid microcarcinoma and the adjacent capsule on preoperative US can predict the presence of extrathyroidal extension, thus helping the surgeon plan the extent of surgical resection [31].

US is superior to computed tomography (CT) scanning in evaluating the presence of abnormal cervical lymph nodes. Cervical lymph nodes can be involved in 20%–50% of patients with differentiated thyroid cancer; more specifically, in those individuals with papillary thyroid cancer [32, 33]. Preoperative US can identify suspicious cervical lymphadenopathy in 20%–31% of cases of thyroid cancer [4].

Recently, evidence suggests that preoperative US may alter the planned surgical procedure in cases where newly discovered multifocal thyroid cancer with regional metastasis may alert the surgeon to perform a total thyroidectomy with extended neck dissection [24, 25]. Preoperative US can identify suspicious cervical lymphadenopathy in 20%–31% of cases of thyroid cancer, thereby potentially altering the extent of and overall surgical approach in these patients [25, 34, 35].

This imaging modality allows for the early detection of nonpalpable cervical lymph node metastasis prior to thyroidectomy in patients with FNA-proven or suspected thyroid cancer that otherwise might have been missed intraoperatively, thereby minimizing the risk for persistent disease [25, 34, 35]. Typical US features of metastatic lymph nodes include hypoechogenicity, rounded appearance, irregular borders, macro- or microcalcifications, loss of the fatty hilus, and increased size [6].

Ultrasound for Thyroid Cancer Surveillance

US can also be used to monitor for recurrent disease in those patients who have undergone surgical resection for thyroid cancer. In fact, currently US is the most frequently used imaging study for monitoring and evaluating patients treated for thyroid cancer postoperatively. Ultrasound surveillance can detect recurrent disease in the thyroid bed after total thyroidectomy or lobectomy, in a remaining contralateral lobe, or in lateral neck lymph nodes. Malignant lymph nodes are more likely to occur in levels III, IV, and VI than in level II [36]. In low-risk patients who have undergone total thyroidectomy without subsequent radioiodine therapy or thyroid lobectomy alone, US may serve as the main surveillance modality postoperatively because this imaging study is highly sensitive in detecting cervical lymph node metastasis [37]. US can be performed without discontinuing thyroid hormone therapy, thus avoiding hypothyroidism, and without administration of recombinant thyroid-stimulating hormone, both of which are required for radioiodine imaging. Therefore, low-risk patients with negative thyroglobulin measurements treated for papillary thyroid cancer may only require periodic US, thus eliminating the need for traditional radioactive iodine imaging. Following surgery and/or radioiodine therapy, US evaluation of the thyroid bed and central and lateral cervical nodal basins can be performed at 6 and 12 months, and then periodically thereafter, depending on the patient's risk for recurrent disease [25, 37]. Further studies are needed to address the cost-effectiveness of US as compared to other imaging modalities in the post-treatment surveillance of certain thyroid cancer patients.

Postoperative US is also useful in guiding surgical planning for reoperations for recurrent thyroid cancer. US has the potential to detect recurrent thyroid cancer when thyroglobulin levels are elevated but radioiodine or positron emission tomography (PET) scans fail to detect it. Localization and mapping of such disease assists in surgical planning of thyroid cancer recurrence, which enables a tailored compartmental neck dissection according to the node basins involved [35, 38]. Surgical management of nonpalpable cervical recurrent disease may prove difficult because of extensive scar formation and fibrosis resulting from previous surgery [35, 38]. US-guided tattooing of recurrent thyroid cancer in the neck using charcoal has been shown to be a safe and effective method in the localization and removal of nonpalpable recurrent disease in patients after previous neck procedures [39].

Ultrasound Guided Therapies for Thyroid Nodules

During the past couple decades, various minimally invasive treatments, directed towards office-based management of symptomatic nodules, without requiring general anesthesia, and with negligible damage to the skin and cervical tissues, have been proposed. Today, US-guided percutaneous ethanol injection and thermal ablation with laser or radiofrequency have been thoroughly evaluated, and are accessible procedures in specialized centers. In clinical practice, relapsing thyroid cysts are effectively managed with percutaneous ethanol injection treatment [40]. For solid nonfunctioning thyroid nodules that grow or become symptomatic, trained operators may safely induce, with a single session of laser ablation treatment or radiofrequency ablation, a 50% volume decrease and, in parallel, improve local symptoms [40].

In contrast, hyperfunctioning nodules remain best treated with radioactive iodine, which results in a better control of hyperthyroidism, also in the long-term, and fewer side-effects. Currently, minimally invasive treatment is also investigated for achieving local control of small size neck recurrences of papillary thyroid carcinoma in patients who are poor candidates for repeat cervical lymph node dissection. Moreover, minimally invasive treatment may provide palliative management of patients at high risk of surgical complications or for individuals who decline further surgery. Overall, minimally invasive treatment of both benign and malignant foci should still be considered experimental due to limited available prospective data confirming long-term symptomatic relief and/or cure versus reduction of tumor burden [40].

Conclusion

US has become an indispensible diagnostic modality in the evaluation of thyroid nodules for benignity and malignancy. This imaging study is useful in the diagnosis, staging, and post-treatment surveillance of initial and recurrent thyroid cancer. Future developments in US usage may lead to further improvements in its diagnostic accuracy and expanded use.

References

[1] Hegedus L. Clinical practice. The thyroid nodule. *The New England Journal of Medicine* 2004;351(17):1764-1771.

[2] Coleman P, Babb P, Damiecki P, Grosclaude P, Honjo S, Jones J, et al. *Cancer survival trends in England and Wales* 1971-1995. London: Stationery Office; 1999.

[3] Mazzaferri EL. Management of a solitary thyroid nodule. *The New England Journal of Medicine* 1993;328(8):553-559.

[4] Lew JI, Solorzano CC. Use of ultrasound in the management of thyroid cancer. *The Oncologist 2010*;15:253-258.

[5] Papini E, Guglielmi R, Bianchini A et al. Risk of malignancy in nonpalpable thyroid nodules: Predictive value of ultrasound and color-Doppler features. *J Clin Endocrinol Metab* 2002;87:1941–1946.

[6] Marqusee E, Benson CB, Frates MC et al. Usefulness of ultrasonography in the management of nodular thyroid disease. *Ann Intern Med* 2000;133: 696–700.

[7] Méndez W, Rodgers SE, Lew JI et al. Role of surgeon-performed ultrasound in predicting malignancy in patients with indeterminate thyroid nodules. *Ann Surg Oncol* 2008;15:2487–2492.

[8] Jabiev AA, Ikeda MH, Reis IM et al. Surgeon-performed ultrasound can predict differentiated thyroid cancer in patients with solitary thyroid nodules. *Ann Surg Oncol* 2009;16:3140 –3145.

[9] Kim EK, Park CS, Chung WY et al. New sonographic criteria for recommending fine-needle aspiration biopsy of nonpalpable solid nodules of the thyroid. *AJR Am J Roentgenol* 2002;178:687– 691.

[10] Moon WJ, Jung SL, Lee JH et al. Thyroid Study Group, Korean Society of Neuro- and Head and Neck Radiology. Benign and malignant thyroid nodules: US differentiation—multicenter retrospective study. *Radiology* 2008; 247:762–770.

[11] Bonavita JA, Mayo J, Babb J et al. Pattern recognition of benign nodules at ultrasound of the thyroid: Which nodules can be left alone? *AJR Am J Roentgenol* 2009;193:207–213.

[12] Asteria C, Giovanardi A, Pizzocaro A, Cozzaglio L, Morabito A, Somalvico F, Zoppo A. US-elastography in the differential diagnosis of benign and malignant thyroid nodules. T*hyroid* 2008;18: 523–531.

[13] Dighe M, Bae U, Richardson ML, Dubinsky TJ, Minoshima S, Kim Y. Differential diagnosis of thyroid nodules with US elastography using carotid artery pulsation. *Radiology* 2008;248:662–669.

[14] Dighe M, Kim J, Luo S, Kim Y. Utility of the ultrasound elastographic systolic thyroid stiffness index in reducing fine-needle aspirations. *J Ultrasound Med* 2010;29:565–574.

[15] Hoang JK, Lee WK, Lee M, Johnson D, Farrell S. US Features of thyroid malignancy: Pearls and pitfalls. *Radiographics* 2007;27:847–860. discussion 61–65.

[16] Luo S, Kim EH, Dighe M, Kim Y. Thyroid nodule classification using ultrasound elastography via linear discriminant analysis. *Ultrasonics* 2011;51:425–431.

[17] Lyshchik A, Higashi T, Asato R, Tanaka S, Ito J, Mai JJ, Pellot-Barakat C, Insana MF, Brill AB, Saga T, Hiraoka M, Togashi K. Thyroid gland tumor diagnosis at US elastography. *Radiology* 2005;237:202–211.

[18] Ophir J, Cespedes I, Ponnekanti H,YazdiY, Li X. Elastography:A quantitative method for imaging the elasticity of biological tissues. *Ultrason Imaging* 1991;13:111–134.

[19] Park SH, Kim SJ, Kim EK, Kim MJ, Son EJ, Kwak JY. Interobserver agreement in assessing the sonographic and elastographic features of malignant thyroid nodules. *AJR Am J Roentgenol* 2009;193: W416–W423.

[20] Rago T, Santini F, Scutari M, Pinchera A, Vitti P. Elastography: New developments in ultrasound for predicting malignancy in thyroid nodules. *J Clin Endocrinol Metab* 2007;92:2917–2922.

[21] Kim MH, Luo S, Ko SH, Bae JS, Lim J, Lim DJ, Kim Y. Thyroid nodule parameters influencing performance of ultrasound elastography using intrinsic compression. *Ultrasound in Med & Biol* 2015; S0301-5629(15)00328-2.

[22] Lim DJ, Luo S, Kim MH, Ko SH, Kim Y. Interobserver agreement and intraobserver reproducibility in thyroid ultrasound elastography. *AJR Am J Roentgenol* 2012;198:W1–W6.

[23] Davies L, Welch HG. Increasing incidence of thyroid cancer in the United States, 1973–2002. *JAMA* 2006;295:2164 –2167.

[24] Milas M, Stephen A, Berber E et al. Ultrasonography for the endocrine surgeon: A valuable clinical tool that enhances diagnostic and therapeutic outcomes. *Surgery* 2005;138:1193–1201.

[25] Kouvaraki MA, Shapiro SE, Fornage BD et al. Role of preoperative ultrasonography in the surgical management of patients with thyroid cancer. *Surgery* 2003;134:946 –955.

[26] Danese D, Sciacchitano S, Farsetti A et al. Diagnostic accuracy of conventional versus sonography-guided fine-needle aspiration biopsy of thyroid nodules. *Thyroid* 1998;8:15–21.

[27] Carmeci C, Jeffrey RB, McDougall IR et al. Ultrasound-guided fine-needle aspiration biopsy of thyroid masses. *Thyroid* 1998;8:283–289.

[28] Seiberling KA, Dutra JC, Gunn J et al. Ultrasound-guided fine needle aspiration biopsy of thyroid nodules performed in the office. Laryngoscope 2008;118:228 –231.

[29] Bhatki AM, Brewer B, Robinson-Smith T et al. Adequacy of surgeonperformed ultrasound-guided thyroid fine-needle aspiration biopsy. *Otolaryngol Head Neck Surg* 2008;139:27–31.

[30] Park JS, Son KR, Na DG et al. Performance of preoperative sonographic staging of papillary thyroid carcinoma based on the sixth edition of the AJCC/UICC TNM classification system. *AJR Am J Roentgenol* 2009;192:66–72.

[31] Kwak JY, Kim EK, Youk JH et al. Extrathyroidal extension of welldifferentiated papillary thyroid microcarcinoma on US. *Thyroid* 2008;18:609–614.

[32] Scheumann GF, Gimm O, Wegener G et al. Prognostic significance and surgical management of locoregional lymph node metastases in papillary thyroid cancer. *World J Surg* 1994;18:559 –568.

[33] Chow SM, Law SC, Chan JK et al. Papillary microcarcinoma of the thyroid—prognostic significance of lymph node metastasis and multifocality. *Cancer* 2003;98:31– 40.

[34] Solorzano CC, Carneiro DM, Ramirez M et al. Surgeon-performed ultrasound in the management of thyroid malignancy. *Am Surg* 2004;70:576–580; discussion 580–582.

[35] Stulak JM, Grant CS, Farley DR et al. Value of preoperative ultrasonography in the surgical management of initial and reoperative papillary thyroid cancer. *Arch Surg* 2006;141:489–496.

[36] Leboulleux S, Girard E, RoseMet al. Ultrasound criteria of malignancy for cervical lymph nodes in patients followed up for differentiated thyroid cancer. *J Clin Endocrinol Metab* 2007;92:3590 –3594.

[37] Torlontano M, Crocetti U, Augello G et al. Comparative evaluation of recombinant human thyrotropin-stimulated thyroglobulin levels, 131I wholebody scintigraphy, and neck ultrasonography in the follow-up of patients with papillary thyroid microcarcinoma who have not undergone radioiodine therapy. *J Clin Endocrinol Metab* 2006;91:60–63.

[38] Lee L, Steward DL. Sonographically-directed neck dissection for recurrent thyroid carcinoma. *Laryngoscope* 2008;118:991–994.

[39] Kang TW, Shin JH, Han BK et al. Preoperative ultrasound-guided tattooing localization of recurrences after thyroidectomy: Safety and effectiveness. *Ann Surg Oncol* 2009;16:1655–1659.

[40] Papini E, Pacella CM, Misischi I, Guglielmi R, Bizzarri G, Dossing H, Hegedus L. The advent of ultrasound-guided ablation techniques in nodular thyroid disease: Towards a patient-tailored approach. *Best Practice & Research Clinical Endocrinology & Metabolism* 2014;28:601-618.

In: Thyroid Nodules
Editor: Marsha Vasquez

ISBN: 978-1-63483-592-3

Chapter III

Pediatric Thyroid Nodules and Well Differentiated Thyroid Carcinoma: Risk Factors, Evaluation, and Management

Jennifer Osipoff, MD, FAAP and Melissa Pawelczak, MD
Stony Brook Children's
Hofstra North Shore-LIJ School of Medicine, Hempstead, NY, US

Abstract

While thyroid carcinoma is rare in the pediatric and adolescent population, it is important for pediatricians and other health care providers to assess for risk of malignancy and order appropriate diagnostic tests in conjunction with consultation with an endocrinologist when confronted with a thyroid mass in a young patient. This chapter will provide the reader with a framework from which to develop a differential diagnosis and initial evaluation plan for such a child or adolescent presenting with a thyroid nodule; identify the risk factors associated with malignant thyroid nodules; appreciate the limitations of ultrasonography and fine-needle aspiration biopsy in the assessment of a thyroid nodule; recognize the risk factors inherent in surgical thyroidectomy; and understand the role of radio-active iodine treatment in the management of thyroid carcinoma. General pediatricians, sub-specialists, and parents alike will welcome the summary of the current state of knowledge in the management of pediatric thyroid nodules and well differentiated thyroid carcinoma (WDTC).

Introduction

Compared to adults, palpable thyroid nodules in children and teenagers are relatively rare with an estimated prevalence of 0.2-1.4% [1]. However, despite their lower occurrence, studies estimate 9 to 50% (mean 26.4%) of thyroid nodules in the pediatric population are cancerous, significantly higher than the estimated 10-14% of lesions in adults [2]. Overall, thyroid carcinoma is rare in the pediatric and adolescent population, with an annual incidence of 2.25/100,000 in individuals under age 20 [3]. While thyroid cancers account for only 1%–2% of childhood malignancies, such growths are the third most common solid tumor in children [4]. WDTC comprise the vast majority of pediatric thyroid malignancies, with papillary carcinoma (PTC) and follicular carcinoma (FTC) accounting for 80-95% and 5-15% of these tumors respectively [5, 6]. Given the risk for cancerous lesions, it is essential that all pediatric health care providers be familiar with how to examine for thyroid nodules, assess for potential risk factors for malignancy, and when it is appropriate to refer the child to a specialist. In turn, the specialists, including but not limited to (pediatric) endocrinologists, head and neck surgeons, and oncologists must be intimately familiar with the necessary screening and diagnostics tests as well as the appropriate surgical and post-operative management of these patients.

Assessing the Patient

The Physical Exam

While traditionally the examiner is taught to palpate the thyroid gland from behind the patient [7]. it has been the experience of these authors that in the case of the pediatric patient the exam may be easier if directly facing the child. The child is asked to tilt his/her head back, allowing for inspection of the neck. The examiner should run his/her fingers down the midline feeling for the ridges of the thyroid and cricoid cartilage. Seemingly misleading, the thyroid gland sits at the level of the cricoid cartilage and the examiner should move his/her fingers laterally to palpate the thyroid until feeling the medial edge of the sternocleidomastoid muscles. Unless a goiter is present, it may be difficult to appreciate the thyroid tissue. A mass in this region is concerning for a thyroid nodule.

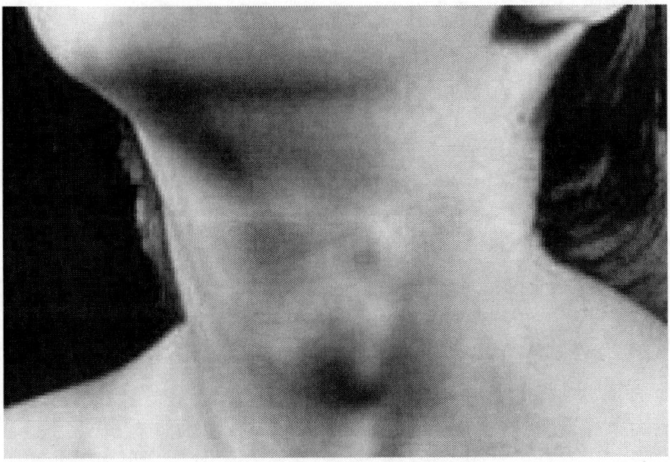

Figure 1. A patient with marked cervical lymphadenopathy prior to diagnosis with PTC.

Thyroid nodules in pre-pubertal children have a higher risk of malignancy. A thyroid nodule found in a male younger than 15 years old has the greatest chance of being malignant.

The size of a nodule has little predictive value into whether or not it will ultimately prove to be malignant. Factors concerning for malignancy include: 1) being irregularly shaped 2) masses that are firm and painless 3) if the lesion is fixed to the surrounding tissue and 4) associated regional lymphadenopathy (Figure 1).

Painful masses or those with overlying erythematous skin changes are more likely to be suppurative thyroiditis and should be treated appropriately. Occasionally thyroid carcinoma will present as peripheral non-tender lymph node enlargement without a detectable thyroid nodule on exam. Therefore it is imperative to consider thyroid malignancy in the differential diagnosis of all painless cervical lymphadenopathy, especially if the patient has any of the risk factors mentioned below.

The Patient and Family Interview

As most children with ultimately proven malignant thyroid nodules are clinically and biochemically euthyroid, the initial detection of a thyroid mass is usually an incidental exam finding and should prompt additional questioning to help assess the risk of cancer. Ionizing radiation to the head or neck, such as that used in in the past for treatment of acne, head and neck hemangiomas, and tonsillar hypertrophy, is an independent risk factor for the development of thyroid malignancies. While the aforementioned treatments are not typically used today, many protocols for childhood cancer (e.g., Hodgkin lymphoma and central nervous system tumors) do employ irradiation of the head and neck. Screening for thyroid malignancies should be a routine part of the post-treatment follow-up care for these oncology patients. It is imperative to keep in mind that several decades may pass between the radiation exposure and the development of thyroid cancer emphasizing the need for long term surveillance. Currently there is no data available to determine whether or not screening beyond an annual physical exam impacts long term outcomes in these high risk individuals [8].

Questioning where the child has lived throughout the course of his/her life is also essential. Iodine deficiency, though rare in the United States, has been linked to thyroid cancers and it is crucial to determine if the child originates from an area of endemic iodine deficiency.

A family history of thyroidectomies, thyroid malignancies, or other cancers suggests that the child with the thyroid nodule has a genetic predisposition to the development of thyroid carcinoma. Genetic disorders such as APC-Associated Polyposis (e.g., familial adenomatoid polyposis and Gardener's syndrome) [9], the Carney complex [10], the DICER1 syndrome [11, 12], the PTEN Hamartoma Tumor Syndrome [13-15], and Werner Syndrome [16] are all associated with the development of both benign and malignant thyroid nodules. Similar to the aforementioned high risk oncology patients, unless a palpable nodule is appreciated, physical exam alone is recommended for most children born into these kindreds (8). However, for those with confirmed PTEN or APC mutations routine ultrasound screening is recommended [13, 14, 17].

The review of systems is invaluable in stratifying the risk of malignancy and guiding the work-up. One should assess for symptoms of pain in the region, excess thyroid hormone production, thyroid hormone deficiency, and structural abnormalities. If the patient complains of pain or tenderness over the nodule, hemorrhage into a cyst, thyroid abscess, or an inflammatory process should be considered before malignancy. Tachycardia, tremulousness, diarrhea—symptoms consistent with hyperthyroidism-- increases the likelihood that the thyroid mass is a solitary toxic adenoma or a multinodular goiter, both of which are unlikely to be malignant, but should be removed surgically. Caution must be exhibited when a patient presents with a discrete thyroid mass and symptoms of hypothyroidism, such as cold intolerance or constipation. While the nodule in this situation likely represents inflammatory change in the setting of Hashimoto's thyroiditis, there is literature that suggests that the presence of chronic lymphocytic thyroiditis raises the risk for thyroid cancers [18]. Though rare in young patients with thyroid nodules, voice changes, symptoms of airway compression, or rapid growth of the lesion are worrisome for malignancy.

The Workup

Laboratory Tests

Thyroid stimulating hormone (TSH), thyroxine (T4), and, in cases where hyperthyroidism is suspected, triiodothyronine (T3), levels should be obtained. Prior to any surgical intervention, medical management should be used to optimize thyroid function. Although laboratory tests cannot differentiate a benign process from a malignant one, a suppressed TSH is suggestive of a hyperfunctioning nodule. An evaluation for a toxic adenoma or a multinodular goiter should be undertaken in this situation via an iodine-123 thyroid uptake and scan. Anti-thyroid peroxidase antibodies and anti-thyroglobulin antibodies should also be measured as their presence may increase the risk of malignancy (see above).

Calcitonin is used to screen for medullary thyroid carcinoma (MTC), a cancer which originates from the parafollicular or C-cells of the thyroid gland, in adults. Sporadic MTC is rare in the pediatric population and MTC usually clusters in families. The 2015 ATA Task Force argues that given the low prevalence of sporadic MTC and the lack of validated reference ranges for pediatrics, further studies need to be undertaken before calcitonin can be recommended as a routine screening test in the work up of pediatric thyroid nodules [8]. The inherited forms of MTC, either as part of multiple endocrine neoplasia (MEN) or familial MTC, are due to an activating mutation in the

RET gene. If suspected, genetic analysis should be performed. Additionally, evaluation for a concomitant pheochromocytoma with a 24 hour urinary catecholamine collection is imperative as this tumor would need to be removed prior to thyroid surgery to prevent hypertensive crisis.

Ultrasound

Ultrasound of the thyroid gland and regional lymph nodes offers a radiation-free method of characterizing thyroid nodules and assessing for local metastasis. Although carcinoma cannot be diagnosed from an ultrasound alone, certain radiographic findings are more commonly seen in malignant lesions (see Figures 2 and 3). Ultrasound can detect changes in the cervical lymph nodes, a finding that greatly increases the likelihood of malignancy. Those these findings have been well validated in adult populations, until recently were being applied to the pediatric population without supporting data. However, a recent meta-analysis of the use of ultrasound for detection of thyroid cancer in the pediatric population exclusively confirmed that internal calcifications and lymph node changes carry the highest likelihood ratio for thyroid cancer [19]. Furthermore they found that the description of taller than wide nodules was not used in the articles they reviewed; therefore they concluded that this may not be something seen commonly in pediatric thyroid malignancies but should still be considered a risk for malignancy in children. Ultrasound is also able to detect non-palpable thyroid nodules, which carry the same risk for malignancy as palpable nodules. Studies have found that if there are multiple nodules, the individual risk of malignancy in each nodule decreases but the overall cancer risk remains the same as a patient with a solitary nodule.

Fine Needle Aspiration Biopsy (FNAB)

FNAB is considered the gold-standard for pre-operative diagnosis of thyroid nodules in adults. Three recent studies [1, 5, 20] investigated the utility of FNAB in pediatrics and each concluded that FNAB is a highly sensitive test that should be utilized in all pediatric patients presenting with a thyroid nodule. A meta-analysis of 12 studies of pediatric FNAB found the pooled sensitivity to be 82% and specificity 91% [20]. Assuming 20% of pediatric thyroid nodules are malignant, the meta-analysis determined the accuracy, positive predictive value, and negative predictive value of FNAB to be 83.6%, 55.3%, and 98.2% respectively. FNAB under ultrasound guidance allows for non-palpable nodules to be biopsied and decreases the chance of a non-diagnostic biopsy; given the inherent difficulties in obtaining a biopsy in children the ATA task force supports that all pediatric FNAB be conducted using ultrasound guidance [8].

Hypoechoic lesions
Intranodal Microcalcifications
Intranodular central vascularization
Lesions that are more tall than wide
Lymph nodes alterations: irregular margins, increased size, lack of echogenic hilum, calcifications, & irregular vascularity

*There is considerable overlap between ultrasound findings of benign and malignant lesions.

Figure 2. Ultrasound Findings Concerning for Malignancy*.

Benign FNAB results, such as a colloid nodule, can prevent unnecessary surgery. Atypical, malignant or indeterminate cytology results guides the appropriate surgical intervention.

FNAB is not without limitations. The diagnostic yield is dependent on the person obtaining the biopsy collecting a sufficient sample and the pathologist reading the cytology report. It is difficult to obtain a diagnostic sample from nodules less than 1cm. However, given the increased risk of malignancy in the pediatric population, given the appropriate clinical context and ultrasound findings, FNAB should still be considered if less than 1 cm. Although FNAB can identify PTC, follicular adenomas and carcinomas cannot be distinguished by FNAB alone and require surgical pathology to determine if the lesion invades the thyroid capsule. The small neck size of young children and the need for sedation in most pediatric patients pose additional challenges in obtaining an FNAB. Adverse events, such as hemorrhage or abscess formation, are extremely rare following a FNAB.

Surgical Management

While a consensus for early, prophylactic total thyroidectomy in children at risk for inheritable MTC has been long standing [21], until the recent publication of the ATA task force [8] the optimal surgical management of WDTC in the pediatric and adolescent population remained controversial. The 2015 guidelines however clearly state "for the majority of children, total thyroidectomy is recommended" [8]. Despite a slightly higher surgical risk, total thyroidectomy allows radioiodine scanning and thyroglobulin levels to be used to detect metastases and disease recurrence (see next section). The majority of patients with PTC have microscopic foci of PTC in the contralateral thyroid lobe. Removing the entire gland eliminates these foci as potential sites of disease recurrence. This decreases the need for a "completion thyroidectomy," a second surgery associated with higher rates of surgical complications [6]. The extent to which cervical lymph nodes should be surgically explored is beyond the scope of this chapter.

It is imperative that any surgeon performing thyroid surgery on a pediatric patient have a great deal of experience in this area. The ATA task force states that the surgeon would ideally perform at least 30 such procedures annually [8]. The task force emphasizes the need for multidisciplinary pediatric care when such a procedure is performed and recommends that the surgery take place in a hospital that has access to high volume surgeons, endocrinologists, radiologists, nuclear medicine specialists, anesthesiologists, and pediatric intensivists. The most frequent complications of total thyroidectomy, permanent hypoparathyroidism with resultant hypocalcemia and permanent laryngeal nerve paralysis causing voice changes and dysphagia, occur in approximately 2% and 1% of patients respectively [22]. Performing the surgery at a center that offers all that is recommended by the ATA task force has been associated with lower complication rates, shorter hospital stays, and decreased costs [8].

Post-Operative Management

Assessing for Residual Disease and Metastases

The American Thyroid Association uses the Tumor Nodes Metastases (TNM) to identify patients at risk of persistent cervical disease and help determine which patients should undergo postoperative staging for the distant metastasis screening. Based upon their TNM classification, patients are stratified into the ATA Pediatric Low-Risk group (disease confined to the thyroid gland and /or incidental evidence of minimal microscopic disease to lymph nodes in the central neck), Intermediate-Risk or High-Risk (these two groups are at greater risk for persistent regional or distant metastasis due to the presence of extensive, extra-thyroidal invasion or metastasis) [8].

Compared to adults, pediatric patients with thyroid cancer have a higher incidence of lymph node involvement and distant metastases at initial presentation.

Per the 2015 American Thyroid Association Guidelines for Children with Thyroid Nodules and Differentiated Thyroid Cancer, children that fall into the ATA Pediatric Low-Risk category may be initially assessed and followed with a TSH-stimulated thyroglobulin (Tg) alone. Thyroglobulin, a protein used in the production of endogenous thyroid hormone, is produced exclusively by the thyroid and thyroid cancer thereby allowing it's measurement to be useful in disease surveillance for WDTC.

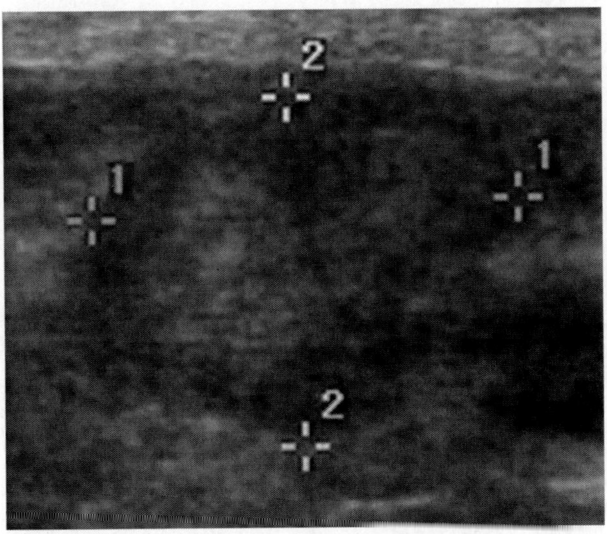

Figure 3. Ultrasound finding of a thyroid nodule. Note the internal calcifications. The patient was ultimately diagnosed with PTC and underwent a total thyroidectomy followed by radioactive iodine ablation.

As TSH stimulation causes thyroglobulin to rise, levels should be measured after levothyroxine withdrawal or following rhTSH injection. Disease recurrence or residual thyroid remnant is suggested by Tg levels above 8 ng/mL while hypothyroid or above 2 ng/mL after rhTSH administration. Levels should be undetectable when TSH is not elevated. As antithyroglobulin antibodies are present in up to 20-25% of patients with

WDTC and interfere with the Tg assay rendering Tg levels uninterpretable [8] such antibodies should be routinely screened.

ATA Pediatric Intermediate-and High-Risk patients should have a TSH-stimulated Tg and, additionally, a diagnostic whole body scan (WBS) to assess for evidence for persistent disease [8].

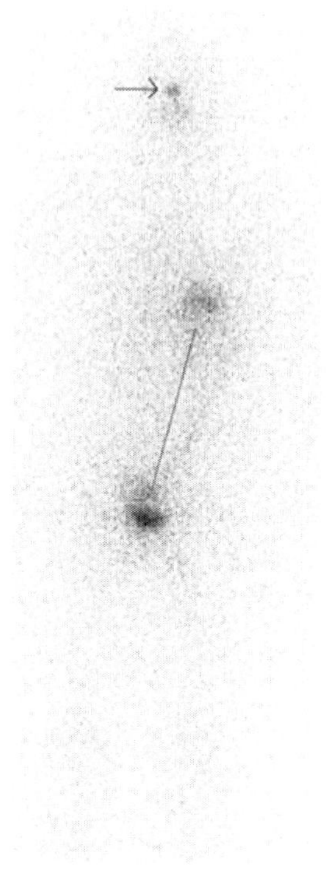

Figure 4. Example of a radioactive iodine whole body scan. Patient had a total thyroidectomy for PTC. At the time of the scan the patient's TSH was 39 mIU/L. The blue arrow points to remnant tissue in the thyroid bed. The red arrow is pointing to the kidney and bladder. As the radioactivity is excreted through the urine, this is a normal finding on a whole body scan. There is no evidence of metastases.

As WDTC cells typically concentrate iodine, radioiodine whole-body scanning (WBS) is a useful tool in the identification of metastases and remnant tissue in the thyroid bed postoperatively. WBS must be performed after surgical treatment of WDTC as iodine avid thyroid tissue concentrates radioiodine more readily than malignant cells. To maximize radioiodine uptake, prior to the WBS, high iodine content foods should ideally be eliminated from patients' diets for two weeks and radiographic contrast should be avoid in the prior 2 to 3 months. As TSH must be above 30 mIU/L to facilitate uptake [23-25] levothyroxine should be held prior to WBS. Most children will achieve the desirable TSH level once levothyroxine is withheld for greater than 2 weeks [26]. Triiodothyronine supplementation can be considered in children who exhibit sensitivity to hypothyroid symptoms or for whom thyroid hormone replacement is withheld for more than 3 weeks (8). Use of recombinant human TSH (rhTSH) avoids the need for withdrawal of thyroid hormone therapy and in adults may result in as much as 1/3 lower absorbed radiation activity to the blood [27]. Although data in children are limited, use of rhTSH raises the TSH to the desired level and appears to be safe making such therapy a useful alternative in instances where endogenous elevation of TSH is not possible or should be avoided for medical reasons [8]. After confirming TSH elevation, WBS is undertaken 24 to 72 hours following administration of I-123 using a scintillation camera designed to capture emitted radiation from the ingested isotope (Figure 4).

I-123 is the preferred isotope for WBS as it provides superior imaging quality and leads to lower absorbed tissue radiation doses than I-131 [28, 29]. Surgical re-exploration is warranted for residual tumor or significant tissue in the thyroid bed.

TSH Suppression

TSH stimulation of WDTC cells may result in increased growth. Therefore, depriving the cancerous cells of TSH via suppression with levothyroxine is a goal of WDTC treatment. The degree of suppression is also under debate as there are no data in children comparing outcomes of differing suppression treatment strategies [8]. As per the 2015 ATA Management guidelines, the desired level of TSH suppression should be determined by ATA Pediatric risk level and current disease status. TSH suppression should be maintained in children with known or suspected persistent disease. The benefits of TSH suppression need to be balanced against its potential risks. Long term complications of excessive levothyroxine include headaches, insomnia, difficulty concentrating, and problems with skeletal maturation and mineralization. TSH can be normalized to the low-normal range after an appropriate period of surveillance in children with no evidence of disease [8].

I-13I Therapy

All children with WDTC should have continued surveillance with monitored TSH suppression. While I-131 therapy has been the mainstay of treatment in children with persistent disease or metastases, the indolent, slow growing nature of WDTC in children creates the therapeutic challenge of avoiding the potential complications of therapy over many years while preventing disease-related morbidity and obtaining disease free survival. The most recent guidelines state that I-131 is indicated for treatment of nodal or other locoregional disease that is not amenable to surgery in addition to distant metastases that are known or presumed to be avid to iodine (8). Some experts also recommend I-131 treatment for children with extensive regional nodal involvement or with T3 tumors [30, 31]. Although complete remission may be achievable with I-131 therapy for many patients with pulmonary metastases, administration of multiple doses may be required [32]. As I-131 therapy has potential inherent risks, particularly with the administration of multiple doses, and pediatric patients with WDTC and pulmonary metastases have an overall favorable prognosis, a balance must be achieved between the desire for a disease free state and the potential harms of therapy. The acute risks of I-131 therapy are well described and include sialadenitis, dental caries, stomatitis, xerostomia, ocular dryness, and nasolacrimal duct obstruction [33, 34]. Gonadal damage has also been reported in both genders as well as acute bone marrow suppression [35-37]. Of great concern, a few studies have shown an increase in secondary malignancies and an overall increase in mortality in patients of all ages treated with I-131 [38]. It is unknown whether the increase in second malignancies follows a threshold does of I-131 or may occur after any amount of I-131. In addition, for patients with lung metastases, a retained I-131 activity of greater than 80 mCi (3Gbq) results in a significant risk for I-131 induced pulmonary fibrosis. As pediatric patients have a potential long lifespan following diagnosis of WDTC and there are a paucity of long term follow up studies of pediatric patients treated with I-131, practitioners should use caution when treating children with I-131 and the potential risks and benefits of therapy should be explained to patients and their families.

For children in whom I-131 is indicated, dosing is commonly determined by either whole body dosimetry or empiric dosing. No data exists comparing the efficacy, long term outcomes or safety of either approach in children. Children should be well hydrated prior to administration of I-131 to support clearance of the radioisotope. A WBS should be obtained 4-7 days after I-131 therapy. If new lesions are identified, SPECT/CT may be useful in defining the precise location of the focal uptake [8].

Long Term Follow-Up

Neck ultrasound and monitoring of non-stimulated Tg with concurrent assessment for the presence of antibodies to thyroglobulin are the preferred method for assessing recurrence or disease progression. Once patients are in remission, an undetectable TSH-stimulated Tg is a reliable predictor of continued disease free state. Repeat TSH-stimulated antibodies are not indicated if the TSH-suppressed Tg is detectable (indicating continued disease) or if a previous TSH-stimulated Tg was undetectable. Neck ultrasound should be performed at least 6 months after initial surgery. Thereafter, ATA Pediatric Intermediate- and High-Risk patients should be followed every 6-12 months and ATA Pediatric Low-Risk patients should be followed annually. After 5 years, follow up should be tailed to the individual based on recurrence risk. In children previously treated with I-131 with no evidence of persistent disease, a WBS may be considered to confirm the absences of iodine avid disease 1-2 years after initial therapy [8]. As the pediatric patient grows older, it is important to arrange for appropriate transition of care to an adult endocrinologist.

Prognosis

Fortunately, despite more frequent advanced disease at diagnosis than adults, pediatric and adolescent patients with WDTC have an excellent prognosis with higher survival rates than their adult counterparts with less invasive disease. The overall survival rate is approximately 99% at 10 years, 95% at 20 years, and 90% at 30 years. However, this population is at an increased risk of disease recurrence. Historically, the progression free survival rates are markedly lower with 65-70% at 5 years, 61% at 10 years, and 46% at 20 years [6, 39]. Thyroid capsule invasion, soft tissue invasion, positive surgical margins, presence of distant metastases at diagnosis, and presentation at less than 15 years old have all been cited as risk factors for disease recurrence [39]. The impact of more aggressive surgical treatment, use of radioiodine, and TSH suppression remains to be seen. As recurrence has been reported as long as 40 years after initial therapy, children with WDTC should be followed for life [8].

Conclusion

WDTC in children poses unique diagnostic and therapeutic challenges. While the incidence of the disease is overall rare in the pediatric population, when identified, thyroid nodules are much more likely to be malignant in children than in adults. Once WDTC is diagnosed in children, considering the overall excellent prognosis, providers must balance the potential harmful risks of therapy against the disease process itself. The approach to surgical intervention has been largely standardized. However, the need for and dosing of I-131 remains controversial. Long term prospective studies are needed to assess the outcomes of children with WDTC treated with and without radioactive iodine.

References

[1] Corrias A, Einaudi S, Chiorboli E, Weber G, Crino A, Andreo M, et al. Accuracy of fine needle aspiration biopsy of thyroid nodules in detecting malignancy in childhood: comparison with conventional clinical, laboratory, and imaging approaches. *J Clin Endocrinol Metab*. 2001 Oct;86(10):4644-8.

[2] Niedziela M. Pathogenesis, diagnosis and management of thyroid nodules in children. *Endocr Relat Cancer*. 2006 Jun;13(2):427-53.

[3] Institute NC. SEER Cancer Statistics Review, 1975-2005. Bethesda [cited 2008]; Available from: http://seer.cancer.gov/csr/1975_2005.

[4] Dinauer C, Francis GL. Thyroid cancer in children. Endocrinol Metab Clin North Am. 2007 Sep;36(3):779-806, vii.

[5] Bargren AE, Meyer-Rochow GY, Sywak MS, Delbridge LW, Chen H, Sidhu SB. Diagnostic utility of fine-needle aspiration cytology in pediatric differentiated thyroid cancer. *World J Surg*. Jun;34(6):1254-60.

[6] Parisi MT, Mankoff D. Differentiated pediatric thyroid cancer: correlates with adult disease, controversies in treatment. *Semin Nucl Med*. 2007 Sep;37(5):340-56.

[7] Zitelli BaD, HW. Atlas of Pediatric Physical Diagnosis. Fifth ed. Philadelphi: Mosby Elsevier; 2007.

[8] Francis G, Waguespack, Steven G., Bauer, Andrew J., Angelos, Peter, Benvenga, Salvatore, Cerutti, Janete, Dinauer, Catherine A., Hamilton, Jill K., Hay, Ian D., Luster, Markus, Parisi, Marguerite T., Rachmiel, Marianna, Thompson, Geoffrey, Yamashita, Shunichi. Management Guidelines for Children with Thyroid Nodules and Differentiated Thyroid Cancer The American Thyroid Association Guidelines Task Force on Pediatric Thyroid Cancer. *Thyroid*. 2015.

[9] Septer S, Slowik, V, Morgan, R, Dai, H, Attard, T. Thyroid Cancer Complicating Familial Adenomatous Polyposis: Mutation Spectrum of At-Risk Individuals. *Hereditary Cancer in Clinical Practice*. 2013;11.

[10] Bertherat J, Horvath A, Groussin L, Grabar S, Boikos S, Cazabat L, et al. Mutations in regulatory subunit type 1A of cyclic adenosine 5'-monophosphate-dependent protein kinase (PRKAR1A): phenotype analysis in 353 patients and 80 different genotypes. The Journal of clinical endocrinology and metabolism. [Research Support, N.I.H., Extramural Research Support, N.I.H., Intramural Research Support, Non-U.S. Gov't]. 2009 Jun;94(6):2085-91.

[11] de Kock L, Sabbaghian N, Soglio DBD, Guillerman RP, Park BK, Chami R, et al. Exploring the Association Between DICER1 Mutations and Differentiated Thyroid Carcinoma. *J Clin Endocr Metab*. 2014 Jun;99(6):E1072-E7.

[12] Doros L, Schultz KA, Stewart DR, Bauer AJ, Williams G, Rossi CT, et al. DICER1-Related Disorders. In: Pagon RA, Adam MP, Ardinger HH, Wallace SE, Amemiya A, Bean LJH, et al. editors. GeneReviews(R). Seattle (WA)1993.

[13] Smith JR, Marqusee E, Webb S, Nose V, Fishman SJ, Shamberger RC, et al. Thyroid nodules and cancer in children with PTEN hamartoma tumor syndrome. The Journal of clinical endocrinology and metabolism. [Case Reports]. 2011 Jan;96(1):34-7.

[14] Ngeow J, Mester J, Rybicki LA, Ni Y, Milas M, Eng C. Incidence and clinical characteristics of thyroid cancer in prospective series of individuals with Cowden and Cowden-like syndrome characterized by germline PTEN, SDH, or KLLN alterations. The Journal of clinical endocrinology and metabolism. [Research Support, N.I.H., Extramural Research Support, Non-U.S. Gov't Research Support, U.S. Gov't, Non-P.H.S.]. 2011 Dec;96(12):E2063-71.

[15] Pilarski R, Burt R, Kohlman W, Pho L, Shannon KM, Swisher E. Cowden syndrome and the PTEN hamartoma tumor syndrome: systematic review and revised diagnostic criteria. *J Natl Cancer Inst.* [Review]. 2013 Nov 6;105(21):1607-16.

[16] Lapunzina P. Risk of tumorigenesis in overgrowth syndromes: a comprehensive review. *Am J Med Genet C Semin Med Genet.* [Review]. 2005 Aug 15;137C(1):53-71.

[17] Papathomas TG, Gaal J, Corssmit EP, Oudijk L, Korpershoek E, Heimdal K, et al. Non-pheochromocytoma (PCC)/paraganglioma (PGL) tumors in patients with succinate dehydrogenase-related PCC-PGL syndromes: a clinicopathological and molecular analysis. European journal of endocrinology / *European Federation of Endocrine Societies.* [Case Reports]. 2014 Jan;170(1):1-12.

[18] Hung W. Solitary thyroid nodules in 93 children and adolescents. a 35-years experience. *Horm Res.* 1999;52(1):15-8.

[19] Al Nofal A, Gionfriddo MR, Javed A, Haydour Q, Brito JP, Prokop LJ, et al. Accuracy of thyroid nodule sonography for the detection of thyroid cancer in children: systematic review and meta-analysis. *Clinical endocrinology.* 2015 Apr 2.

[20] Stevens C, Lee JK, Sadatsafavi M, Blair GK. Pediatric thyroid fine-needle aspiration cytology: a meta-analysis. *J Pediatr Surg.* 2009 Nov;44(11):2184-91.

[21] Kloos RT, Eng C, Evans DB, Francis GL, Gagel RF, Gharib H, et al. Medullary thyroid cancer: management guidelines of the American Thyroid Association. *Thyroid.* 2009 Jun;19(6):565-612.

[22] Bargren AE, Meyer-Rochow GY, Delbridge LW, Sidhu SB, Chen H. Outcomes of surgically managed pediatric thyroid cancer. *J Surg Res.* 2009 Sep;156(1):70-3.

[23] Rachmiel M, Charron M, Gupta A, Hamilton J, Wherrett D, Forte V, et al. Evidence-based review of treatment and follow up of pediatric patients with differentiated thyroid carcinoma. Journal of pediatric endocrinology & metabolism : *JPEM.* [Review]. 2006 Dec;19(12):1377-93.

[24] Spoudeas HA. Paediatric Endocrine Tumours Multi-Disciplinary Consensus Statement of Best Practice from a Working Group Convened Under the Auspices of the The British Society of Paediatric Endocrinology & Diabetes and the United Kingdom Children's Cancer Study Group. West Sussex, United Kingdom2005.

[25] Dinauer CaFG. Thyroid Cancer in Children. *Endocrinology and Metabolism Clinics of North America* 2007. p. 779-806.

[26] Kuijt WJ, Huang SA. Children with differentiated thyroid cancer achieve adequate hyperthyrotropinemia within 14 days of levothyroxine withdrawal. *The Journal of clinical endocrinology and metabolism.* 2005 Nov;90(11):6123-5.

[27] Hanscheid H, Lassmann M, Luster M, Thomas SR, Pacini F, Ceccarelli C, et al. Iodine biokinetics and dosimetry in radioiodine therapy of thyroid cancer: procedures and results of a prospective international controlled study of ablation after rhTSH or hormone withdrawal. *J Nucl* Med. [Multicenter Study Randomized Controlled Trial Research *Support*, Non-U.S. Gov't]. 2006 Apr;47(4):648-54.

[28] Cohen JB, Kalinyak JE, McDougall IR. Clinical implications of the differences between diagnostic 123I and post-therapy 131I scans. *Nucl Med Commun.* [Clinical Trial]. 2004 Feb;25(2):129-34.

[29] Urhan M, Dadparvar S, Mavi A, Houseni M, Chamroonrat W, Alavi A, et al. Iodine-123 as a diagnostic imaging agent in differentiated thyroid carcinoma: a comparison with iodine-131 post-treatment scanning and serum thyroglobulin measurement. *Eur J Nucl Med Mol Imaging.* [Comparative Study Controlled Clinical Trial]. 2007 Jul;34(7):1012-7.

[30] Chow SM, Law SC, Mendenhall WM, Au SK, Yau S, Mang O, et al. Differentiated thyroid carcinoma in childhood and adolescence-clinical course and role of radioiodine. *Pediatr Blood Cancer.* [Comparative Study]. 2004 Feb;42(2):176-83.

[31] Jarzab B, Handkiewicz-Junak D, Wloch J. Juvenile differentiated thyroid carcinoma and the role of radioiodine in its treatment: a qualitative review. *Endocr Relat Cancer.* [Research Support, Non-U.S. Gov't Review]. 2005 Dec;12(4):773-803.

[32] Pawelczak M, David R, Franklin B, Kessler M, Lam L, Shah B. Outcomes of children and adolescents with well-differentiated thyroid carcinoma and pulmonary metastases following (1)(3)(1)I treatment: a systematic review. Thyroid : *official journal of the American Thyroid Association.* [Review]. 2010 Oct;20(10):1095-101.

[33] Goolden AW, Kam KC, Fitzpatrick ML, Munro AJ. Oedema of the neck after ablation of the thyroid with radioactive iodine. *Br J Radiol.* [Case Reports]. 1986 Jun;59(702):583-6.

[34] Kloos RT, Duvuuri V, Jhiang SM, Cahill KV, Foster JA, Burns JA. Nasolacrimal drainage system obstruction from radioactive iodine

therapy for thyroid carcinoma. *The Journal of clinical endocrinology and metabolism.* 2002 Dec;87(12):5817-20.

[35] Sawka AM, Lakra DC, Lea J, Alshehri B, Tsang RW, Brierley JD, et al. A systematic review examining the effects of therapeutic radioactive iodine on ovarian function and future pregnancy in female thyroid cancer survivors. Clinical endocrinology. [Evaluation Studies Research Support, Non-U.S. Gov't Review]. 2008 Sep;69(3):479-90.

[36] Sawka AM, Lea J, Alshehri B, Straus S, Tsang RW, Brierley JD, et al. A systematic review of the gonadal effects of therapeutic radioactive iodine in male thyroid cancer survivors. Clinical endocrinology. [Research Support, Non-U.S. Gov't]. 2008 Apr;68(4):610-7.

[37] Verburg FA, Hanscheid H, Biko J, Hategan MC, Lassmann M, Kreissl MC, et al. Dosimetry-guided high-activity (131)I therapy in patients with advanced differentiated thyroid carcinoma: initial experience. *Eur J Nucl Med Mol Imaging*. 2010 May;37(5):896-903.

[38] Rubino C, de Vathaire F, Dottorini ME, Hall P, Schvartz C, Couette JE, et al. Second primary malignancies in thyroid cancer patients. British journal of cancer. [Comparative Study Research Support, Non-U.S. Gov't]. 2003 Nov 3;89(9):1638-44.

[39] Grigsby PW, Gal-or A, Michalski JM, Doherty GM. Childhood and adolescent thyroid carcinoma. *Cancer*. 2002 Aug 15;95(4):724-9.

In: Thyroid Nodules
Editor: Marsha Vasquez

ISBN: 978-1-63483-592-3

Chapter IV

Cancer Thyroid Nodule: Knowing Is Doing

Maria Concetta Trovato**, MD, PhD
Department of Clinical and Experimental Medicine,
University of Messina, Messina, Italy

Abstract

In the last decade, the incidence of malignant thyroid cancer has increased worldwide. This escalation has derived either from a precocious individualization of small carcinomas or a major occurrence of large carcinomas. As a counterweight to early diagnosis, the mortality has not decreased but has rather increased.

Epithelial malignant cancers of the thyroid emerge as nodules set up by two different cellular types such as follicular and parafollicular cells, namely C cells. The former, producing thyroid hormones, develop either well differenced thyroid carcinomas (WDTC) or anaplastic carcinomas; while the latter, secreting calcitonin, make up medullary thyroid carcinomas (MTC).

WDTC account for 90% of all thyroid cancers and are classified as papillary thyroid cancer (PTC) (80–85%), follicular thyroid cancer (FTC) (10–15%) and Hurtle cell carcinoma (HCC) (3–5%). Overall, WDTC

* Address: Policlinio Universitario, via Gazzi, Messina, Italy; Phone: 331 0902212590, Email: mariatrovato@tin.it, trovatom@unime.it

have good prognosis with disease free survival close to 95% for PTC and 80% for FTC. ATC are occurring in 1 to 2% of thyroid cancers and display a poor prognosis. MTC include the remaining 5 to 9% of thyroid cancer and show a relatively poor prognosis. Multiple gene mutations and rearrangements harbour in thyroid cancers. Affected genes include RET, BRAF, PI3KCA, RAS, MET and Galectin. Chromosomal rearrangements involve especially chromosome 7 and 10.

Morphology of cells already plays a main role for identification of cancer in nodules and to drive patients toward appropriate treatments.

The latest is that molecular medicine may work in diagnostic identification of thyroid cancers as a marker and therefore, could modify the flow chart for management of thyroid nodules.

Introduction

Mostly, the neoplasms of thyroid come out as nodular formations. Thyroid nodules (TN) affect 10-18 million of USA individuals, increase with age, are more common in women in respect to men (4.3% versus 1.2%), are detected in 10% of adult population and in 50% of autopsy studies and may appear either by a single nodule or multiple diffuse lumps [1, 2]. A malignant proliferation is found in 7% of thyroid solitary nodules while in multinodular glands, the possibility to encounter a cancer is around 9% [3].

In the last three decades the incidence of thyroid cancers (TC) has continuously increased and this trend is recorded on every continent [4]. In women, TC is the fifth most common cancer and in Italy the second most frequent cancer in women under 45 years old [5, 6]. Therefore, the efforts to improve the knowledge about TN and risk factors determining the malignant transformation of nodules are urgent. The common tool for both clinicians and pathologists is to make up clinical pathological classifications able to individualize cancerous nodules in the large context of TN and in parallel to offer the best therapeutic strategy to patients differentiating medical from surgical TC.

Surgery therapy is broadly employed to cure TN, nonetheless, acceptable classifications of thyroid nodular lesions, combining histological and clinical information adequate to address the patients to surgery, is still a goal yet to be achieved. This is confirmed by recent epidemiological data reporting that 42-77% of nodules removed are diagnosed benign and surgical excision could be evitable [7, 8].

However, these statistical data have to be read through the concept of nodular thyroid disease that may induce clinical symptoms either as a lump or by overproduction of thyroid hormones [9]. In general, TN may be defined independently from biological malignancy as neck masses that are able to induce compressive clinical symptoms [10]. Therefore, a lobectomy is an adequate therapeutic strategy for benign TN causing symptoms such as compression, hoarseness, shortness of breath or difficulty swallowing. In addition, a total, or near total thyroidectomy may be recommended for patients with enlarged multinodular goiters or hyperthyroidism [10, 11]. By evaluating biological malignancy of TN, the surgery solution may be considered for nodules measuring >1.5 cm or for aggressive cancers [10, 11].

A simplistic, but practical, cataloging of TN share benign from malignant types and subdivided the latter in well-differentiated (WDTC) and undifferentiated carcinomas (UDTC). At large, the total removal of the thyroid gland is recommended for UDTC while a limited resection is indicated for WDTC and therefore, when definitive histological diagnosis is made a complete resection may follow [12, 13]. However, these surgical approaches to TC is controversial, because of the risks of reoperation to complete thyroidectomy and so, many surgeons tend to consider it necessary to remove the whole gland even in the presence of WDTC [12]. Further, several surgeons have drawn attention to the high rate of complications following useless thyroidectomy and advocate its use in more limited circumstances [8].

The problem to find a helpful classification of TN, to be used by clinicians and pathologists in common practice diagnostic to address patients toward adapted therapeutic choices, is furthermore complicated by pre-operatory diagnosis made up of TN by fine needle aspiration (FNAB) [14]. Cyto-pathological examination represents the gold standard to distinguish benign from malignant thyroid lesions in pre-operatory stage and then, the best method to adequately alert patients toward surgery [15]. In fact, FNAB individualizes 60%-75% of benign lesions, 3%-6% of malignant nodules and it is non-diagnostic in only 5%-8% of nodules. The major problem of thyroid FNAB is the category of indeterminate samples including 15-30% of nodules aspirated [10, 16, 17]. In the absence of valid indications, very often these indeterminate cases receive unnecessary surgery. To overcome this impasse of FNAB, in the near past, cytology features data have been associated with standard technique results, such as ultrasound examination (US), Doppler examination, imaging CT scan, MRI or PET scanning, and biochemical markers [18]. In this way, the use of different investigations has increased the sensitivity and specificity of FNAB, reducing the percentage of indeterminate cases. At present, there is the proposal to combine FNAB with molecular investigation recognizing TC genetic markers [10, 20]. On the basis of genetic rearrangements occurring in TC, cancerous markers are currently being tested to combine with FNAB to isolate TC from TN.

Two genetic pathways are being investigated to serve as genetic markers of thyroid carcinogenesis: firstly, genetic alterations occurring in RET, BRAF, PI3KCA, RAS, MET and Galectin genes; secondly, rearrangements of 7 and 10 chromosomes [20-29].

The aim of this study was an overview of TN classifications to associate with risk factors and diagnostic markers of TC in order to individualize sensitive diagnostic procedures adequate for clear therapeutic addresses for both benign and malignant lesions.

From Morphological to Flow Chart of Thyroid Nodules

Morphology of TN may be individualized either *in situ* or by microscopy.

In situ, TN are defined by radiological investigations as discrete lesions within the thyroid gland that may be distinct from the surrounding thyroid parenchyma [10]. By US features, TN may appear as solid (STN) or with cystic component (CTN) when the cystic formation accounts for 10% of the total volume [11, 12].

The signatures indicating benignancy of STN include ovoid shape, isoechogenicity, smooth margin, and peripheral vascularity. Whereas, in STN borderline appear US images of hypoechogenicity, central vascularity and macrocalcifications. Lastly, the malignancy of STN is individualized through marked hypoechogenicity, speculated margins, microcalcifications and taller-than-wide shapes [11, 12].

The benign characteristics of CTN consist of configuration, concentric or eccentric with a blunt angle, smooth free margins, peripheral or any vascularity, spongiform features or additional cysts in the solid component, and isoechogenicity.

In contrast, US malignant signs of CTN encompass from eccentric configuration of the main solid or cystic component with an acute angle, microcalcifications, macrolobulation or irregularity of borders, perinodular infiltration to centripetal vascularity [11, 12].

By microscopy, TN are classified on the basis of four criteria such as cytogenetic, architectural, cytomorphological and histopathogenetic.

Cytogenetic Criteria

Cytogenetic criteria refer to the cell type from which TN originates. In thyroid glands two major types of epithelial cells functionally distinct, such as follicular and parafollicular or C-cells are recognized. Therefore, TN and TC may be set up by follicular cells or C-cells. The nodular formations containing follicular cells retain the ability to convert iodine into thyroxine and triiodothyronine while TC of C-cells secrete calcitonin. On the basis of cytogenetic criteria, TN are denominated follicular and TN with hyperplasias of C cells, while TC are distinct in follicular and medullary thyroid carcinomas (MTC), respectively. These distinctions have practical diagnostic vantages to isolate and monitor TN and TC lesions. Specifically, thyroid scintigraphy is the nuclear medicine examination that uses the ability of follicular cells to produce thyroid hormone to evaluate thyroid tissue [30]. Therefore, scintigraphic examination is able to provide clinical information on functional status of TN, TC or metastatic TC cells. Furthermore, serum dosages of TSH, thyroid hormones and Calcitonin are indicated to detect the presence of TC metastasis in post thyroid surgery stage [31].

Architectural Criteria

Architectural criteria evaluate the construction of nodular lesions. Principally, by architectural findings, follicular TN may be distinct in hyperplasic (HTN) and neoplastic (NTN) and the latter in benign and malignant TN [32], respectively. The sign distinguishing HTN from NTN is the recognition of a true fibrous capsule built through production of connective tissue and surrounding the perimeter of NTN. In opposition, HTN show a false fibrous capsule arranged through phenomena of compression on interstitial connective fibers resulting from the increase of follicular cells. The difference between the true and false capsule may be individualized in the production of connective tissue occurring only in the true capsule [9]. Supplementary, the true capsule is also the sign distinguishing benign TN from malignant. This is because in malignant nodular lesions the capsule is broken by infiltration of malignant follicular or C-cells while the capsule appears uncompromised in benign TN [9]. Vascular invasion is included among signs showing bias among adenomas and carcinomas because it appears only in malignant TN [9].

According to cytogenetic and architectural criteria, the World Health Organization (WHO) has classified primary thyroid tumors in epithelial and non epithelial, and both categories in benign or malignant, respectively [33] (Table 1).

Table 1. WHO Classification (Reference [33])

1. Epithelial tumours
1.1 Benign
1.1.1 Follicular adenoma
1.1.2 Others
1.2 Malignant
1.2.1 Follicular carcinoma
1.2.2 Papillary carcinoma
1.2.3Medullary carcinoma (C-cell carcinoma)
1.2.4 Undifferentiated (anaplastic) carcinoma
1.2.5 Others
2. Non-epithelial tumours
3. Malignant lymphomas
4. Miscellaneous tumours
5. Secondary tumours
6. Unclassified tumours
7. Tumour-like lesions

Benign tumors consisting of follicular cells are called follicular adenomas (FA) while the equivalent malignant forms are subdivided in follicular (FTC), papillary (PTC) and anaplastic (ATC) thyroid carcinomas, respectively. Curable PTC and FTC are the more recurrent histotypes accounting a frequency of 66% and 12%, respectively. Aggressive ATC appears less frequent and comprise 1-2% of all thyroid cancers [34].

The WHO classification has the great vantage of specificity but also the disadvantage of a low sensitivity. In fact, by using the WHO classification it is possible to design unequivocally the origin of TC retaining the practical use of supplying adequate information to monitor advanced cancer. Additionally, the distinction of benign from malignant tumors could further clarify diagnostic, therapeutic and prognostic addresses. However, the clinical practice contradicts this mismatch between diagnosis and prognosis because of TC with intermediate biological behaviour including the hyalinizing trabecular tumors [35]. On the other hand, the detection of PTC microcarcinoma, referred to as incidentaloma, during autopsy, remains a category to uncertain prognostic categorization [36].

Cytomorphological Criteria

Cytomorphological criteria takes two factors into account: firstly, the growth cellular pattern by which follicular and C cells are distributed in TN; secondly, morphologic changes of cytoplasm and nucleus appearing in TN of follicular cells. Both follicular and C cell types grow through papillary and solid patterns, while follicular cells uniquely dispose to construct microfollicular, macrofollicular or cystic formations. The modifications of cytoplasm emerging in follicular cells are designed such as oncocytic, clear, squamous and mucinous changes and appear in both benign and malignant lesions (Figure 1).

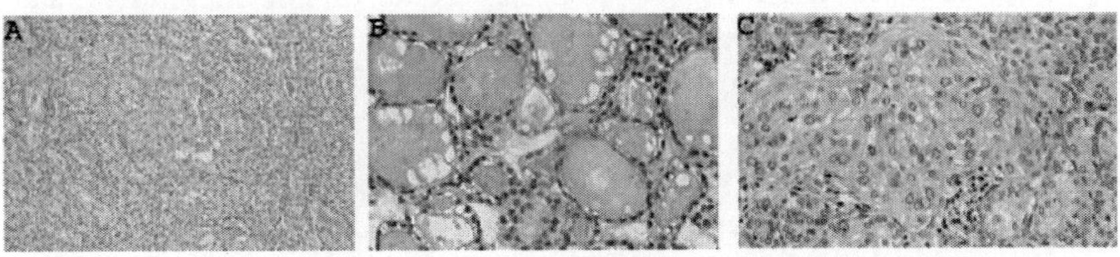

Figure 1. Nuclear and cytoplasmatic modifications of follicular cells appearing either in benign or malignant follicular lesions. A. Oncocytic, B. clear, C. squamous changes, respectively.

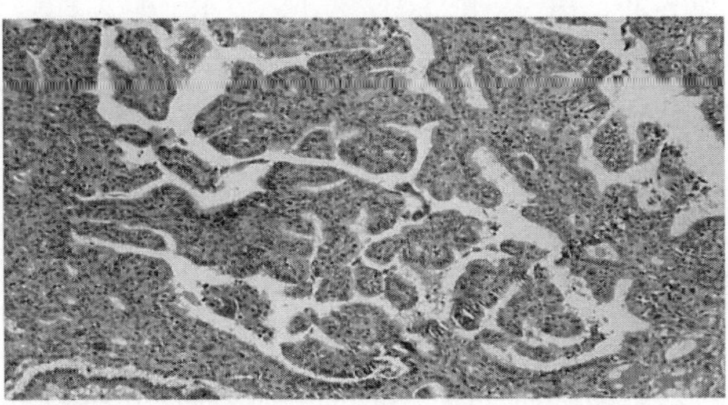

Figure 2. Nuclear modification namely, ground glass or "Orphan Annie's eyes," emerging in papillary thyroid carcinoma, only.

Conversely, the modification of nucleus indicated as ground glass or "Orphan Annie's eyes" occur exclusively in PTC (Figure 2). On the basis of cytomorphological criteria, follicular TN are histologically stratified in colloid nodules (CN), including goiters and thyroditis, FA and carcinomas. CN are detected in 42-77% of TN, FA in 15-40% and carcinomas in 8-17% [32].

Conforming to cytomorphological criteria the classification adopted by the Armed Forces Institute of Pathology (AFIP) has been compiled (Table 2) [37].This scheme is slightly different from the WHO classification in that it gives priority to cellular morphology and incorporates special tumor types and subtypes, namely "variants."

The AFIP classification has the vantage to conjunct both diagnostic and prognostic responses by overcoming the criteria of unique types of malignancy opposite to benignity. In practice, follicular malignant TC are subdivided into three categories such as well-differentiated (WDTC), poorly differentiated (PDTC) and undifferentiated carcinomas (UDTC). WDTC are curable and show a good prognosis, while PDTC, including insular form, and UDTC, including ATC types, have mid-term and poor prognosis, respectively [38]. WDTC are frequent accounting for 90% of all TC and are distinct in PTC and FTC [9]. Disease free survival is close to 95% for PTC and 80% for FTC [9]. The main diagnostic element sharing PTC from FTC is recognition of nuclear alterations occurring in PTC cells and indicated as ground glass appearance, overlapping, pseudoinclusions and nuclear grooves [37]. The variants of PTC are due to the papillary pattern of growth and the size of follicular cells [37]. By papillary pattern, PTC are classified in classic, follicular, encapsulated, diffuse, sclerosing and solid/trabecular variants, respectively [37]. By morphology of follicular cell covering papillae, PTC include oxyphilic cell and tall and columnar cell variants [37].

Against this background of the AFIP classification, that includes PTC among WDTC, there is the prognosis of PTC. In fact, PTC has not unequivocally a good prognosis and for almost 20 years the debate on different prognosis of PTC variants is still ongoing [38, 39, 37] (Table 3). A good prognosis is unanimously recognized in PTC variants namely, microcarcinoma, encapsulated and macrofollicular, respectively. The prognosis is variable for oxyphilic cell, follicular, solid and trabecular PTC types.

Diffuse sclerosing as well as tall and columnar cell PTC variants are still, to this day, "guarded" for their evolution and under observation by the scientific community for a clear prognostic response [38, 39, 37].

Table 2. AFIP Classification (Reference [37])

PRIMARY TUMORS
1. Epithelial tumours
A. Tumors of follicular cells
    Benign: Follicular adenoma (conventional, variants*)
    Malignant: carcinoma
    Differentiated: follicular carcinoma
        papillary carcinoma (conventional, variants**)
        Poorly differentiated (insular carcinoma, others)
        Undifferentiated or anaplastic
B. Tumors of C-cells (and related neuroendocrine cells)
    Medullary carcinoma
    others
C. Tumors of follicular and C-cells
    mixed medullary-follicular carcinoma
2. Sarcomas
3. Malignant lymphoma (and related hematopoietic neoplasms)
4. Miscellaneous neoplasms
SECONDARY TUMORS
TUMOR-LIKE LESIONS

*oncocytic, clear cell changes, atypical adenoma, hyalinizing trabecular, with bizarre nuclei.

**microcarcinoma, encapsulated, follicular, oncocytic, tall/columnar cell, diffuse sclerosing, solid/trabecular.

On the same line of PTC, the prognosis of WDTC namely FTC cannot be defined completely good because of the FTC variant namely, Hürthle cell tumors [40]. This is a malignant follicular TC because it is composed of follicular cells arranged in follicles, and malignancy is recognized by capsular infiltration and vascular invasion. The cytomorphological diagnostic elements of this variant are oncocytes or Hürthle cells that cover over 75% of TC cellular population. Nevertheless, there is some evidence of natural history of this tumor suggesting to consider oncocytic FTC variant as a separate entity because of a worse prognosis in respect to FTC [40, 41].

In agreement with cytological criteria schemes for cytological examinations of FNAB have been composed (Table 4). Actually, the alterations appearing on thyroid cytological samples are catalogued in four classifications from experiences and reports of American and European thyroid associations from 2007 to 2012 [10, 15-17]. Two lines of conduct have been adopted to compile all cytological classifications: firstly, the quantification of cellular and colloid components appearing on the smears; secondly, nuclear and cytoplasmatic changes of follicular or C cell.

Table 3. Variants of papillary thyroid carcinoma and their prognosis

GOOD
Microcarcinoma
Encapsulated
VARIABLE
Oxyphilic cell
Follicular
Solid/trabecular
GUARDED
Diffuse sclerosing
Tall and columnar cell

This is because cytology is unable to supply information on capsular invasion. The great quality of cytology is in the ability to observe nuclear and cytoplasmatic changes before ordinary therapeutic treatments. By reporting nuclear changes, the cytological examination effortlessly individualizes PTC nodules providing adequate information to address patients to surgery. Conversely, by recognizing oncocytes on cytological smears the presence of potential aggressive lesions may be indicated, only without supplying clear indications for clinician and surgery. This is not connected to the impotence of cytology, on the contrary, this is linked to uncertain knowledge on course of oncoytic lesions.

The main problem of all cytological schemes are lesions made up by follicular cells similar to normal cells of follicles that on histological examination are generically classified as follicular lesions and therefore distinguished in benign and malignant by observation of capsule [10, 15-17]. These lesions are included among cytological categories namely follicular lesion of undetermined significance, follicular neoplasm, suspicion of a follicular neoplasm, suspicion of malignancy. To overcome these problems the amounts of follicular cells and colloid appearing on cytological samples have been considered. This is because of an increase of cellular population that could be detected along hyperplastic, benign and malignant neoplastic lesions while an increase of colloid could be more frequent in benign cystic lesions.

Table 4. Classifications of thyroid cytology

	Bethesda diagnostic category (2007)	American Thyrod Association (2009)	British Thyroid Association (2009)		Italian Thyroid Association (AIT) & Italian Society of Pathology (SIAPEC) (2012)	
I	Non-diagnostic or unsatisfactory	Non-diagnostic/unsatisfactory	Thy1	Non-diagnostic	Tir 1	Not diagnostic
					Tir 1c	Not diagnostic, cystic
II	Benign	Benign	Thy2	Non-neoplastic	Tir 2	Not neoplastic
III	Atypia of undetermined significance or follicular lesion of undetermined significance	Indetermined or suspicious for malignancy	Thy3a	Atypical features present	Tir 3A	Follicular proliferation with low risk
IV	Follicular neoplasm or suspicious for a follicular neoplasm	Indetermined or suspicious for malignancy	Thy3f	Follicular neoplasm suspected	Tir 3B	Follicular proliferation with high risk
V	Suspicious for malignancy	Indetermined or suspicious for malignancy	Thy4	Suspicious of malignancy	Tir 4	Suspicious for malignancy
VI	Malignant	Malignant	Thy5	Diagnostic of malignancy	Tir 5	Malignant

However, these rules are not completely adequate to distinguish benign from malignant since in benign lesions a large cellular population may occur [10, 15-17].

Histopathogenetic Criteria

Histopathogenetic criteria takes into consideration the genesis of TN and factors controlling growth and cellular apoptosis by genetic and epigenetic mechanisms [32]. TN are catalogued such as hyperplastic, neoplastic, colloid, cystic and thyroiditic nodules.

In hyperplastic TN, the proliferation of follicular cells, is kept in line mainly through TSH action developing by TSH receptor (TSHR), cAMP and PKA pathways. Mutation of TSHR is implied in constitutive cAMP overproduction and responsible for overgrowth and hyperfunction of follicular cells. Among the factors involved in proliferation of thyrocytes there are several interleukins, such as IL-6, by which is established a direct link among follicular cells, stromal apparatus and lymphocytes through paracrine and autocrine pathways [42].

In neoplastic TN, the molecular medicine has identified activation of several oncogenes occurring in malignant lesions. The oncogenetic alterations playing major roles in thyroid carcinogenesis are mutations of TSHR and gsp, TRK, that is receptor for NGF; RET/PTC; RAS (encoding Gs proteins that transduces mitogenic signals); BRAF; PI3KCA; c-met, that is receptor for hepatocyte growth factor and Galectin. The more common genetic abnormalities found in PTC are the radio-induced RET/PTC rearrangements and the mutations of BRAF and RAS genes, while the loss of heterozigosity (LOH) on 3p and 7q loci as well as RAS mutations are frequently encountered in FTC. Transition of WDTC towards UDTC is genetically signed by mutation of genomic guardian i.e P53 protein [20].

In the genesis of colloid TN has been supposed a defect of intraluminal reabsorption of hTg to justify the concentrated solution of thyroglobulin (hTg) that is detected in follicles. The experimental data supporting this hypothesis is the regression of follicular hyperplasia towards colloid features by a load of iodine. On the other hand, a defective storage of hTg into polymeric globules that brings about excessive extension of follicles, has been supposed [32].

There are three mechanisms at the root of cystic TN: necrosis, colliquation and angiogenesis. The balance of these processes lead to the formation of "pseudocysts" that occur frequently in TN while true cystic formations are rare. The role of angiogenesis in cystic TN has been evaluated by VEGF/VPF while apoptotic mechanisms have also been advocated [32].

Thyroiditic TN enclose a heterogeneous variety of thyroid diseases in which lymphocytes are present so that the generic indication of "strumite" could be suggested. In fact, lymphocytes are arranged to form lymphatic follicle in Hashimoto's thyroditis disease that may appear as a nodule occuring either in a hyperplastic or normal gland. In addition, lymphocytic infiltration may be associated with PTC and thyroid primitive lymphoma [9].

By histopthogenetic criteria emerge the experimental applications of molecular medicine to FNAB in an effort to improve diagnostic accuracy, so several immunohistochemical and molecular markers have been proposed. Most of them are currently under review on large series and their evaluations, along with their efficient use in routine practice, are offering new diagnostic criteria. The hot point of these prospective studies is to individualize the biological risk of progression for thyroid tumors to address patients towards the better treatment by preventing unnecessary surgery. This is because well-differentiated thyroid cancers progress slowly, produce symptoms only when advanced and rarely cause death [43, 44].

At present, a practice flow chart for management of TN to early individualization of TC have to conjunct morphology and molecular medicine to clinical information. In this way, it is comprehend that an increase of TN size is still the major sign of suspicion for malignancy [45]. Further, by clinical investigation a haemorrhagic thyroid lesion is effectively diagnosed because of rapid increase in size over a few hours, while a benign goitrous TN grows in size over the years and malignancy typically grows in weeks. In the final analysis the size of TN remains the main ratio for surgery indication even for benign TN.

References

[1] Hegedüs L. Clinical practice. The thyroid nodule. *N. Engl. J. Med.* 351(17), 1764–1771, 2004.

[2] Davies L, Welch H.G. Increasing incidence of thyroid cancer in the United States, 1973–2002. *JAMA*. 10;295(18), 2164-267, 2006.

[3] Marqusee E, Benson CB, Frates MC, Doubilet PM, Larsen PR, Cibas ES, Mandel SJ. Usefulness of ultrasonography in the management of nodular thyroid disease. *Ann Intern Med.* 7;133(9):696-700, 2000.

[4] Pellegriti G, Frasca F, Regalbuto C, Squatrito S, Vigneri R. Worldwide increasing incidence of thyroid cancer: update on epidemiology and risk factors. *Cancer Epidemiol.*2013:965212. doi: 10.1155/2013/965212, 2013.

[5] Simard EP, Ward EM, Siegel R, Jemal A. Cancers with increasing incidence trends in the United States: 1999 through 2008. *CA Cancer J Clin*. 62(2):118-28. doi: 10.3322/caac.20141, 2012.

[6] Dal Maso L, Lise M, Zambon P, Falcini F, Crocetti E, Serraino D, Cirilli C, Zanetti R, Vercelli M, Ferretti S, Stracci F, De Lisi V, Busco S, Tagliabue G, Budroni M, Tumino R, Giacomin A, Franceschi S; AIRTUM Working Group. Incidence of thyroid cancer in Italy, 1991-2005: time trends and age-period-cohort effects. *Ann Oncol*, 22(4):957-63. doi: 10.1093/annonc/mdq467, 2011.

[7] Sakorafas GH, Peros G, Farley DR. Thyroid nodules: does the suspicion for malignancy really justify the increased thyroidectomy rates*? Surg Oncol,* 15(1):43-55, 2006.

[8] Bilimoria KY, Zanocco K, Sturgeon C. Impact of surgical treatment on outcomes for papillary thyroid cancer. *Adv Surg,* 42:1-12, 2008.

[9] Trovato M. Chapter VI: New Research Communication on Thyroid Tumor Markers, pagg.69-80, in the book titled "Research Progress in Tumor Markers," Editors Lilly Shafter e Emily Richter (ISBN: 9781604566925), Ed. Nova Science Publishers, Hauppauge New York, USA, 2008.

[10] Cooper DS, Doherty GM, Haugen BR, Kloos RT, Lee SL, Mandel SJ, Mazzaferri EL, McIver B, Pacini F, Schlumberger M, Sherman SI, Steward DL, Tuttle RM. Revised American Thyroid Association management guidelines for patients with thyroid nodules and differentiated thyroid cancer. American Thyroid Association (ATA) Guidelines Taskforce on Thyroid Nodules and Differentiated Thyroid Cancer. Thyroid, 19: 1167214. doi:10.1089/thy.2009.0110, 2009.

[11] Frates MC, Benson CB, Charboneau JW, et al. Management of thyroid nodules detected at US: Society of Radiologists in US consensus conference statement. *Radiology,* 237: 794800. doi:10.1148/radiol.23730 50220, 2005.

[12] Anil G, Hegde A, Chong FHV. Thyroid nodules: risk stratification for malignancy with ultrasound and guided biopsy. *Cancer Imaging*. 11, 209-223 DOI: 10.1102/1470-7330.2011.0030, 2011.

[13] Pacini F, Schlumberger M, Dralle H, Elisei R, Smit JWA, Wiersinga W. European Consensus for the management of patients with differentiated

thyroid carcinoma of the follicular epithelium. *Eur J Endocrinol.*2006; 154, 787-803, 2006.

[14] Borget I, Vielh P, Leboulleux S, Allyn M, Iacobelli S, Schlumberger M, de Pouvourville G. Assessment of the cost of fine-needle aspiration cytology as a diagnostic tool in patients with thyroid nodules. *Am J Clin Pathol.* 129(5):763-771. doi: 10.1309/H86KM785Q9KBWPW5, 2008.

[15] Kocjan G, Feichter G, Hagmar B, Kapila K, Kardum-Skelin I, Kloboves V, Kobayashi TK, Koutselini H, Majak B, Schenck U, Schmitt F, Tani E, Totch M, Onal B, Vass L, Vielh P, Weynand B, Herbert A. Fine needle aspiration cytology: a survey of current European practice. *Cytopathology.* 17(5):219-26, 2006.

[16] Cibas ES, Ali SZ. The Bethesda System for Reporting Thyroid Cytopathology. *Thyroid.* 19(11):1159-165. doi: 10.1089/thy.2009.0274, 2009.

[17] Cochand-Priollet B, Schmitt FC, Tötsch M, Vielh P. European Federation of Cytology Societies' Scientific Committee. The Bethesda terminology for reporting thyroid cytopathology: from theory to practice in Europe. *Acta Cytol.* 55(6):507-11. doi: 10.1159/000334687, 2011.

[18] Tomimori EK, Camargo RYA, Bisi H, Medeiros-Neto G. Combined ultrasonographic and cytological studies in the diagnosis of thyroid nodules *Biochimie*, 81:447-52, 1999.

[19] Schmitt FC, Vielh P. Molecular biology and cytopathology. Principles and applications. *Ann Pathol.* 32(6):e57-63, 444-50. doi: 10.1016/j.annpat.2012.09.210, 2012.

[20] Ruggeri RM, Campennì A, Baldari S, Trimarchi F, Trovato M. What is New on Thyroid Cancer Biomarkers. *Biomark Insights.* 29(3):237-252, 2008.

[21] Prescott JD, Zeiger MA. The RET oncogene in papillary thyroid carcinoma. *Cancer.* 2. doi: 10.1002/cncr.29044, 2015.

[22] Ciampi R, Knauf JA, Rabes HM, Fagin JA, Nikiforov YE. BRAF kinase activation via chromosomal rearrangement in radiation-induced and sporadic thyroid cancer. *Cell Cycle.* 4(4):547-8, 2005.

[23] Kim SK, Woo JW, Lee JH, Park I, Choe JH, Kim JH, Kim JS. Role of BRAF V600E mutation as an indicator of the extent of thyroidectomy and lymph node dissection in conventional papillary thyroid carcinoma. *Surgery.* pii: S0039-6060(15)00439-0. doi: 10.1016/j.surg., 2015.

[24] Ruggeri RM, Vitarelli E, Barresi G, Trimarchi F, Benvenga S, Trovato M. HGF/C-MET system pathways in benign and malignant histotypes of

thyroid nodules: an immunohistochemical characterization. *Histol Histopathol.* 27(1):113-21, 2012.

[25] Ruggeri RM, Vitarelli E, Barresi G, Trimarchi F, Benvenga S, Trovato M. The tyrosine kinase receptor c-met, its cognate ligand HGF and the tyrosine kinase receptor trasducers STAT3, PI3K and RHO in thyroid nodules associated with Hashimoto's thyroiditis: an immunohisto chemical characterization. *Eur J Histochem.* 3;54(2):e24, 2010.

[26] Cecchinelli B, Lavra L, Rinaldo C, Iacovelli S, Gurtner A, Gasbarri A, Ulivieri A, Del Prete F, Trovato M, Piaggio G, Bartolazzi A, Soddu S, Sciacchitano S. Repression of the antiapoptotic molecule galectin-3 by homeodomain-interacting protein kinase 2-activated p53 is required for p53-induced apoptosis. *Mol Cell Biol.* 26(12):4746-57, 2006.

[27] Lavra L, Rinaldo C, Ulivieri A, Luciani E, Fidanza P, Giacomelli L, Bellotti C, Ricci A, Trovato M, Soddu S, Bartolazzi A, Sciacchitano S. The loss of the p53 activator HIPK2 is responsible for galectin-3 overexpression in well differentiated thyroid carcinomas. *PLoS One.* 6(6):e20665. doi: 10.1371/journal.pone.0020665, 2011.

[28] Trovato M, Fraggetta F, Villari D, Batolo D, Mackey K, Trimarchi F, Benvenga S. Loss of heterozygosity of the long arm of chromosome 7 in follicular and anaplastic thyroid cancer, but not in papillary thyroid cancer. *J Clin Endocrinol Metab.* 84(9):3235-240, 1999.

[29] Trovato M, Ulivieri A, Dominici R, Ruggeri RM, Vitarelli E, Benvenga S, Barresi G, Trimarchi F, Brunetti E, Vecchione A, Andreoli M, Sciacchitano S. Clinico-pathological significance of cell-type-specific loss of heterozygosity on chromosome 7q21: analysis of 318 microdissected thyroid lesions. *Endocr Relat Cancer.* 11(2):365-376, 2004.

[30] Elgazzar AH, Alenezi S, Alshammari JM, Ghanem M, Asa'ad S. Value of Oblique View in Nodular Thyroid Disease; Revisiting Fundamentals. *World J Nucl Med.* 14(2):125-27. doi: 10.4103/1450-1147.153911, 2015.

[31] Moeller LC, Führer D. Thyroid hormone, thyroid hormone receptors, and cancer: a clinical perspective. *Endocr Relat Cancer.* 22;20(2):R19-29. doi: 10.1530/ERC-12-0219, 2013.

[32] Salabe GB. Pathogenesis of thyroid nodules: histologic classification? *Biomed Pharmacother.* 55: 39-53, 2001.

[33] Hedinger C, Williams ED, Sobin LH. The WHO histological classification of thyroid tumors: A commentary on the second edition. *Cancer* 63: 908-911, 1989.

[34] Nagaiah G1, Hossain A, Mooney CJ, Parmentier J, Remick SC. Anaplastic thyroid cancer: a review of epidemiology, pathogenesis, and treatment. *J Oncol.* 2011:542358. doi: 10.1155/2011/542358, 2011.

[35] Cheung CC, Boerner SL, MacMillan CM, Ramyar L, Asa SL. Hyalinizing trabecular tumor of the thyroid: A variant of papillary carcinoma proved by molecular genetics. *Am J Surg Pathol* 24: 1622-1626, 2000.

[36] Rosai J, LiVolsi VA, Sobrinho-Simões M, Williams ED. Renaming papillary microcarcinoma of the thyroid gland: The Porto proposal. *Intl J Surg Pathol* 11: 249-251, 2003.

[37] Rosai J, Carcangiu ML, DeLellis RA, Frable W, Tallini G. Tumors of the Thyroid and parathyroid Glands. 21 AFIP Atlas of Tumor Pathology, Series 4, Armed Forces Institute of Pathology, Washington, D.C., 2015.

[38] Sobrinho-Simões M. Tumors of thyroid: A brief overview with emphasis on the most controversial issues. *Curr Diagn Pathol* 2: 15-22, 1995.

[39] Scopa CD. Histopathology of thyroid tumors. An overview. Hormones (Athens). 3(2):100-110, 2004.

[40] Carcangiu ML, Bianchi S, Savino D, Voynick IM, Rosai J. Follicular Hürthle cell tumors of the thyroid. *Cancer* 68: 1944-1953, 1991.

[41] Pappoti M, Torchio B, Grassi L, Favero A, Bussolati G. Poorly differentiated oxyphilic (Hürthle cell) carcinomas of the thyroid. *Am J Surg Pathol* 20: 686-694, 1996.

[42] Ruggeri RM, Barresi G, Sciacchitano S, Trimarchi F, Benvenga S, Trovato M. Immunoexpression of the CD30 ligand/CD30 and IL-6/IL-6R signals in thyroid autoimmune diseases. *Histol Histopathol.* 21(3):249-256, 2006.

[43] Alexander EK, Kennedy GC, Baloch ZW, Cibas ES, Chudova D, Diggans J, Friedman L, Kloos RT, LiVolsi VA, Mandel SJ, Raab SS, Rosai J, Steward DL, Walsh PS, Wilde JI, Zeiger MA, Lanman RB, Haugen BR. Preoperative diagnosis of benign thyroid nodules with indeterminate cytology. *N Engl J Med.* 23;367(8):705-15. doi: 10.1056/NEJMoa1203208, 2012.

[44] Schlumberger M1, Catargi B, Borget I, Deandreis D, Zerdoud S, Bridji B, Bardet S, Leenhardt L, Bastie D, Schvartz C, Vera P, Morel O, Benisvy D, Bournaud C, Bonichon F, Dejax C, Toubert ME, Leboulleux S, Ricard M, Benhamou E; Tumeurs de la Thyroïde Refractaires Network for the Essai Stimulation Ablation Equivalence Trial. Strategies of radioiodine ablation in patients with low-risk thyroid cancer. *N Engl J Med.* 3;366(18):1663-673. doi: 10.1056/NEJMoa1108586, 2012.

[45] Kamran SC, Marqusee E, Kim MI, Frates MC, Ritner J, Peters H, Benson CB, Doubilet PM, Cibas ES, Barletta J, Cho N, Gawande A, Ruan D, Moore FD Jr, Pou K, Larsen PR, Alexander EK. Thyroid nodule size and prediction of cancer. *J Clin Endocrinol Metab.* 98(2):564-570. doi: 10.1210/jc.2012-2968, 2013.

In: Thyroid Nodules
Editor: Marsha Vasquez
ISBN: 978-1-63483-592-3

Chapter V

Medullary Thyroid Cancer

Souha Kallel**, *Moncef Sellami, Firas Maalej, Malek Mnejja, Ilhem Charfeddine, Boutheina Hammami and Abdelmonem Ghorbel

Department of otorhinolaryngology-Head and Neck Surgery
Habib Bourguiba University Hospital,
Sfax, Tunisia

Abstract

The medullary thyroid carcinoma (MTC) is developed from thyroid C cells that secrete calcitonin (CT). MTC accounts for 5–10% of thyroid cancers with a 1–2% incidence in nodular thyroid diseases. It is sporadic in the majority of cases and familial in 20 to 30% of cases. Familial hereditary form is a result of a germline mutation in the *RET* proto-oncogene and can be seen in familial medullary thyroid cancer (FMTC) or as part of the multiple endocrine neoplasia (MEN) syndrome type 2 (2A or 2B). MTC is frequently solitary nodule which is often associated with nodal metastasis. Confirmation is obtained by a high basal calcitonin level which represents specific biological marker. Surgery is the only curative treatment and should consist of total thyroidectomy with central and ipsilateral or bilateral lateral lymph node dissection. A prophylactic

* Phone: +216 53518498. E-mail: souha.kallel@yahoo.fr

thyroidectomy may be performed for at-risk members in the familial form. Radiation therapy does not currently play a significant role in the treatment of MTC. For locally advanced or metastatic MTC, chemotherapy provides little benefit. RET target gene therapy (mainly tyrosine kinase inhibitors) appears as possible promise therapeutic for the future. The prognosis of MTC depends on both the stage of the disease and the extent of the initial surgery.

Definition-Epidemiology

Medullary thyroid cancer (MTC) is a form of thyroid cancer that originates from the parafollicular cells of the thyroid gland. Parafollicular cells (also called C cells) are neuroendocrine cells in the thyroid. These cells originate from neural crest, migrate to the ultimobranchial body, and are incorporated into the thyroid when the ultimobranchial body fuses with the thyroid. They are located adjacent to the thyroid follicles and reside in the connective tissue. These cells are large and have a pale stain compared with the follicular cells.

They are found mostly in the upper and middle parts of the thyroid. C-cells do not secrete thyroid hormone nor do they take up iodine. For this reason, radioactive iodine is not effective in the treatment of the MTC. Instead, the parafollicular cells produce a hormone called calcitonin (CT). The calcitonin hormone contributes in the regulation of calcium metabolism. The serum CT levels are high in patients with MTC and can be useful for diagnosis and post therapeutic monitoring.

MTC represents 5–10% of thyroid cancers and 1–2% incidence in nodular thyroid diseases.

There is two particular forms of MTC:

- The sporadic form (majority of cases). Sporadic MTC is present in the fifth or sixth decade of life and there is a slight female preponderance [1, 2]
- The familial Hereditary form (20-30% of cases). It is a result of a germline mutation in the *ret* proto-oncogene. It can present in isolation (familial medullary thyroid cancer [FMTC]) or as part of the multiple endocrine neoplasia syndrome type 2 (MEN2: MEN2A or MEN2B). MEN2A and FMTC typically present in the third decade of life, and MEN2B usually presents in those younger than age 20.

Clinical Presentation

The symptoms associated with MTC are similar to other forms of thyroid cancer. They include an euthyroid thyroid nodule or multinodular goiter, associated frequently with satellite nodes. This is the most common mode of CMT revelation.

The MTC may be associated with symptoms related to compression (dysphagia, dysphonia, breathing difficulty). Indeed these tumors tend to arise in the posterior thyroid, often invading the surrounding structures [1].

A cervical lymphadenopathy or distant metastases are the mode of revelation in nearly 20% of cases. The most common locations for metastatic MTC are the mediastinum, liver, lungs, and bone.

Flush syndrome and diarrhea remain rare circumstances of diagnosis, and are associated with advanced tumors with a major hypersecretion of CT.

MTC can also present as Cushing syndrome due to the ectopic corticotropin production [3, 4].

There are additional physical features associated with patients who have MEN 2B: an elongated face, nodules on the lips, tongue or on the inside cheeks of the mouth (mucosal neuromas), swollen appearing eyelids or lips, constipation, and scoliosis.

Diagnosis

The routine assay of calcitonin for every thyroid nodule is controversial. Historically, the American Thyroid Association (ATA) MTC guidelines (2009) [5] and European Thyroid Association (ETA) consensus (2006) [6] have been divergent on this matter. Our current literature review showed that the dosage of CT is practiced systematically by most teams [7, 8, 9, 10, 11].

In the case of a uni- or multi-nodular thyroid disease, high CT serum level (≥ 100 pg / ml) is used preoperatively to confirm the diagnosis.

Fine-needle aspiration (FNA) of a thyroid nodule or lymph node allows most frequently the diagnosis, but it was not contributive in nearly half of cases in some series [5, 7, 9].

On cytology, MTC is characterized by the presence of stromal amyloid and the absence of thyroid follicles. FNA cannot always distinguish MTC based on the appearance of the cells alone, so the diagnosis is typically confirmed through the use of immunohistochemistry (positive anti-CT).

Another useful technique that has recently been described is to measure the calcitonin level of the washout fluid from an FNA. This technique appears to be even more sensitive than cytology with immunohistochemistry [12, 13].

Unsuspected MTC can also be found at or after surgery. Macroscopically, MTC is white or gray in color and very firm to palpation. Histologically, MTC is arranged as nests of uniform cells that are characterized by the deposition of stromal amyloid. "C-cell hyperplasia" is defined as 6 C cells per follicle or 50 C cells per low-power field and is often found in patients with hereditary disease. While C-cell hyperplasia is considered a precursor of malignant transformation in hereditary disease, its implication in nonhereditary disease is less well defined.

Currently, most patients with either FMTC or MEN2 are identified by genetic testing of at-risk family members. Family members of patients with a germline mutation of the ret gene have a 50% chance of inheriting the mutation. If patients are identified to be genetic carriers, their lifetime risk for malignancy approaches 100%. The hereditary disease commonly presents with multifocal and bilateral involvement.

Tumor Biological Markers of MTC

Calcitonin

Calcitonin is the principal hormone secreted by the thyroid C cells. Current immunometric assay technique, based on the use of monoclonal antibodies, are specific for the mature monomer CT [14]. The conditions of blood sampling must be observed : fasting, the absence of drug taking potentially responsible of hyper CT (proton pump inhibitors). The basal CT is normally less than 10 pg / ml. For the MTC, there is a good correlation between the CT level and the tumor mass [15]: basal CT concentrations greater than 60 -100 ng/L associated with thyroid nodule are described as highly suggestive / pathognomonic of MTC. A more moderate increase in basal CT concentrations (< 50 pg/ml) may be related to a microscopic MTC but also to a. The C-cell hyperplasia (CCH) that can be due to lymphocytic thyroiditis, benign or malignant thyroid tumor other than the MTC [16, 17, 18] or extra-thyroid diseases such as endocrine tumors, tobacco, chronic renal failure especially in patients on dialysis [19, 20]. In this situation (CT<50 pg / ml), calcitonin stimulation test with pentagastrin (Pg) should be performed.

Calcitonin Stimulation Test

Calcitonin stimulation test with pentagastrin is the most used for diagnosis of MTC. It is required to confirm or refute the need for thyroid surgery in patients with calcitonin values that are 'mildly'elevated.

In healthy adult subjects, peak stimulated CT is less than 30 pg / mL [21, 22]. In CMT, the peak of CT stimulated is usually greater than 100 pg / ml [7, 8, 9]. However, authentic CMT (microcarcinomas) may have a CT response below this value and, conversely, thyroid abnormalities other than MTC (multinodular goiters, colloid adenomas, differentiated thyroid cancers, chronic thyroiditis) may have a response to Pg, (usually <100 pg / ml) [23, 24, 10] reflecting a reactional CCH. In fact, the combination of basal and stimulated CT values is the most sensitive and specific is a good technique for the diagnosis of CMT. A basal CT higher or equal to 30 pg / ml and a CT response to Pg higher or equal to to 200 pg / ml are highly predictive of the diagnosis of CMT with a sensitivity of 90.5% and a specificity of 80.6% [23].

Carcinoembryonic Antigen (CEA)

The CEA is a useful tumor marker in patients with MTC. It is a non-specific marker and less reliable than CT. The CEA levels are inconstantly elevated in patients with MTC (> 50%). A preoperative serum CEA level > 30 ng/ml is highly predictive of the inability to cure a patient with operative intervention [25]. CEA levels >100 ng/ml are highly associated with extensive lymph node involvement and distant metastasis. An increasing CEA level in the presence of a stable calcitonin level can be a sign of dedifferentiation of the tumor and is associated with a worse prognosis.

Familial Forms

Familial forms termed multiple endocrine neoplasia type 2 (MEN 2) are divided into three categories: MEN2A, MEN2B, and FMTC, which are inherited in an autosomal dominant fashion with a high but variable penetrance.

MEN2A (Sipple's Syndrome)

This is the most common MEN2 disorder (60% of MEN2). MTC is associated with pheochromocytoma in up to 50% of cases, and primary hyperparathyroidism in up to 20%–35%. Pheochromocytomas can be screened for using either plasma metanephrines or 24-hour urine collections for catecholamines and metanephrines. Pheochromocytomas should be treated and resected prior to MTC surgery. Hyperparathyroidism is screening for doing serum calcium and parathyroid hormone levels. The disease may manifest as hyperplasia or as a single, enlarged parathyroid gland. Patients should be treated with removal of only the grossly abnormal parathyroid glands.

A few variants of MEN2A are also linked with other disorders like cutaneous lichen amyloidosis at the upper part back. This Cutaneous lichen amyloidosis is linked to mutations on codon 634. A mutation on codon 620 carries a significant risk for developing Hirschsprung disease [26, 27].

MEN2B

This category is less common (affecting 8%–15% of all MEN2 patients). Here, the MTC is associated with pheochromocytoma in up to 50% of cases, and is not associate with hyperparathyroidism. Patients have mucosal neuromas of the lips and tongue and intestinal ganglioneuromas. Chronic constipation and megacolon are also common. Many patients have skeletal deformations such as kyphoscoliosis or lordosis, Marfanoid habitus, everted eyelids, and myelinated corneal nerves [28].

FMTC

The familial medullary thyroid cancer is not associated with other components of the disease. It may be difficult to distinguish FMTC from MEN2A, and identical genetic mutations can causes either disease [29].

As the MTC is often the first manifestation of MEN2A and diagnosis of pheochromocytoma or hyperparathyroidism is often made later. The definition of FMTC is strict. FMTC is a variant of MEN2A with multigenerational MTC without pheochromocytoma or hyperparathyroidism and is revealed after the age of 50 years in multiple family members affected by the disease.

Genetic Testing

The genetic mutation in familial MTC is in the *ret* protooncogene, which is mapped to chromosome 10q11.2 [30]. As *ret* is a proto-oncogene, only a single point mutation is required for malignant transformation. The currently known mutations encode > 95% of cases of hereditary MTC. Among *ret* mutations; there is significant variation in the aggressiveness of the MTC that develops. Thus, currently, *ret* mutations are classified into three groups based on the level of risk for MTC [5, 31]. Level 3 mutations (codon 883, 918, and 922) have the most aggressive course, with metastatic disease presenting in the first years of life. Level 2 *ret* mutations (codon 611, 618, 620, and 634 mutations) are considered high risk for MTC, the risk of MTC appears around the fifth year of life. Level 1 *ret* mutations (codon 609, 768, 790, 791, 804, and 891) are still considered high risk for MTC, but are the lowest risk of the *ret* mutations. MTC in these patients tends to develop later in life and takes on a more indolent course. The most common mutation in MEN-2A is in codon 634, occurring in 80% of patients. The codon most frequently associated with MEN-2B is a codon 918 mutation. The prevalence of family MTC de novo (without known family context) is estimated between 5-16% [31]. Any MTC is potentially a new MEN2 index case, the molecular analysis of the *ret* gene is proposed systematically in any MTC [31, 32, 33]. Once a patient is found to be positive for a *ret* mutation, he or she must be carefully advised regarding the risks to additional family members. At-risk family members need to be identified and should undergo genetic testing; because patients that are identified as *ret* mutation should ideally be offered a prophylactic thyroidectomy prior to the development of MTC.

Treatment

Pre-Operative Staging

Ultrasound examination of the neck should be performed in all patients with MTC. CT chest, dual phase CT liver (Figure 1) or MRI, bone scintigraphy or MRI spine are recommended for systemic staging in patients with extensive neck disease and signs of regional or distant metastases, and in all patients with a serum Ctn level greater than 500 pg/mL [5, 34].

Neither FDG-PET/CT nor F-DOPA-PET/CT recommended in detecting distant metastases

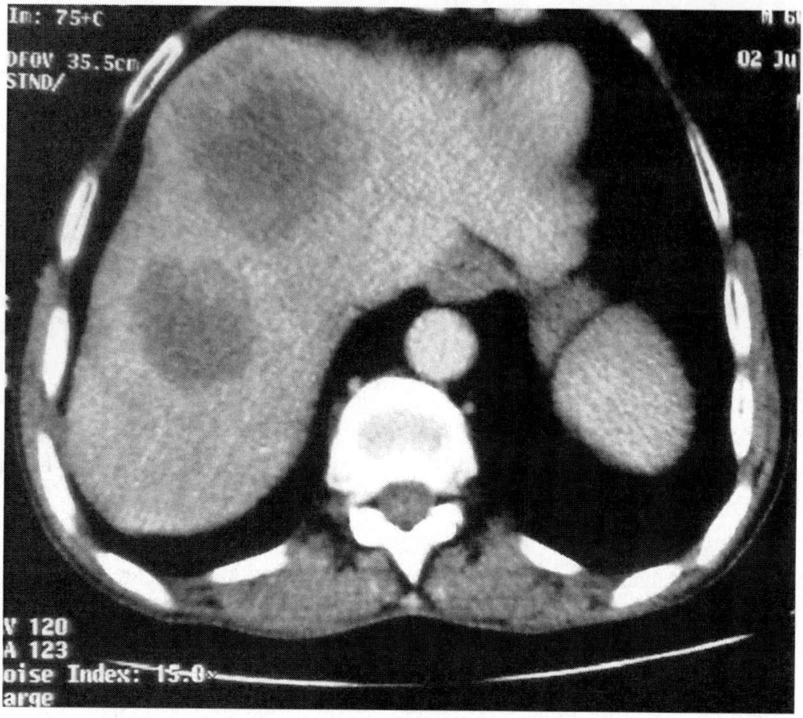

Figure 1. CT scan revealing multiple liver metastasis in a sporadic MTC.

The Initial Surgical Treatment of Patients with MTC

Surgery is the only curative treatment and consist of total thyroidectomy and bilateral central neck dissection [5]. The central neck regional metastasis is found in up to 81% of patients with palpable tumors [35, 36].

The central neck dissection consists of a complete clearing of all lymph nodes and fibrofatty tissues from the level VI compartment. Level VI extends from the hyoid bone superiorly to the sternal notch inferiorly; laterally it is limited by the carotids [37].

For some others, the inferior limit of the dissection being the innominate artery (levels VI and VII) [38].

The need for a prophylactic lateral neck dissection is controversial. Ipsilateral lateral nodal metastases are present in 14%–80% of patients [35, 39] and contralateral lateral nodal metastases in 19%–49% of patients [35, 40].

Lateral neck dissection is recommended for patients with clinical or radiological involved lymph nodes in the lateral compartment, in the presence of central compartment node metastases and in FCMT. Another approach is that ipsilateral lateral neck dissection should be added if the primary tumor is > 1 cm in size [37]. For some teams the lateral neck dissection is systematic [40, 41, 42].

A lateral neck dissection consists of a complete clearing of levels IIa, III, IV and Vb. Routine dissection of levels I, IIb and Va is not required unless there are palpable suspicious nodes at these sites. A contralateral lateral neck dissection should be considered in patients with positive controlateral nodes on US, in bilateral tumors or extensive lymph node involvement ipsilaterally [37]. According to the American Thyroid Association MTC Guidelines [5], when preoperative imaging is positive in the ipsilateral lateral neck compartment but negative in the contralateral neck compartment, contralateral neck dissection should be considered if the basal calcitonin level is greater than 200 pg/mL (Grade C Recommendation).

Even in the presence of distant metastases at presentation, surgery (total thyroidectomy and central compartment node dissection) should be considered to prevent subsequent compromise of the trachea, oesophagus and recurrent laryngeal nerves. These structures should be preserved whenever possible [5, 37].

Prophylactic Thyroidectomy

Prophylactic thyroidectomy is recommended in at-risk patients before the onset of clinically significant disease.

Early prophylactic surgery is effective in reducing both mortality and morbidity.

The possibility of future surgery should be discussed with parents before testing children. In hereditary MTC, there is a strong age-related progression from C-cell hyperplasia to MTC and progression to nodal disease.

- Children with MEN 2B (883, 918, and 922 codons mutation) should undergo prophylactic thyroidectomy within the first year of life [43, 44].

- Children with MEN 2A associated with a 634 codon mutation should undergo thyroidectomy before the age of 5 years [45].
- Prophylactic surgery for MEN 2A gene carriers with other than 634 codon mutations or FMTC, may be delayed, beyond the age of 5 years, provided that the basal calcitonin remains within the normal range [5].

The need for a central node dissection is controversial. Several authors did not indicate neck dissection when preoperative ultrasound is normal with moderately elevated basal calcitonin level.

Radiation Therapy

Radiation therapy does not currently play a significant role in the treatment of patients with MTC. It is indicated in case of important risk of local recurrence. This may be where there is macroscopic residual disease or microscopic residual disease on the background of large volume disease [46, 47].

Radiation therapy is applied to help palliate local disease when surgery is not a feasible option [37]. Radiation therapy may be used to palliate bony metastases.

Systemic Therapy

Patients with metastasis can have severe symptoms from calcitonin excess and may benefit from medical treatment with somatostatin analogs.

Chemotherapy has so far not demonstrated its effectiveness (combinations of doxorubicin, 5-fluorouracil, streptozotocin, dacarbazine, vincristine and cyclophosphamide) with an objective response rate of about 20% and often partial and transient symptomatic improvement, with no survival benefit and a considerable toxicity [48, 49, 50]. Therefore it's not recommended.

A new class of therapies targeting the RET receptor Tyrosine kinase family has been developed because of its role in the pathogenesis of MTC. The tyrosine kinase inhibitors block the abnormal kinase proteins involved in the development and growth of medullary cancer cells. Several kinase inhibitors have been evaluated in phase I and II clinical trials, including axitinib, cabozantinib (XL-184), lenvatinib (E7080), motesanib, pazopanib, sorafenib, sunitinib and vandetanib [51, 52]. Phase II trials showed clear evidence of response in 20-50% of patients. Responses have been stable for periods exceeding 3 years. Two of these agents, vandetanib and cabozantinib have completed phase III clinical trials.

Kinase inhibitors represent currently the most promising option for metastatic CMT and for an inoperable progressive disease. The major side effects of this class of drug include hypertension, nausea, diarrhea, some cardiac electrical abnormalities, and thrombotic or bleeding episodes.

The selective uptake of 131I-mIBG and 111In-octreotide by 30–50% of medullary cancers generated interest in their potential therapeutic use. But usually they have not shown their effectiveness for MTC [53].

Therapies with immunization [54] and radiolabelled molecules have been performed in MTC sometimes with promising results. These treatments cannot be recommended but entry into trials should be considered.

Follow-Up

Thyroid hormone replacement is required after a total thyroidectomy. The follow-up should start 2–3 months postoperatively by obtaining new baseline calcitonin and CEA levels [55, 56]. When calcitonin levels is lower than 10 pg / ml, Calcitonin stimulation test with pentagastrin is indicated for detecting a disease persistence or recurrence. Patients who have undetectable calcitonin levels can be followed with annual measurements of serum calcitonin and CEA. Imaging is indicated when there is a rise in serum markers.

Persistent or Recurrent Disease

It is important to distinguish locoregional, persistent or recurrent disease from distant metastases as the cause of an elevated calcitonin. The surgical resection should be performed if the patient did not have an adequate initial management and for isolated locoregional disease [57]. In case of distant metastases, cervical revision surgery is not indicated and an indication of other treatment should be discussed in a multidisciplinary way. Therefore, if patients develop symptomatic locoregional recurrence, even in the setting of metastatic disease, then they should be offered surgical resection when feasible or external beam radiation therapy when surgery is not possible [58].

In case of residual hyper-CT with an adequate oncological surgery and in the absence of localisable metastasis, scalability of biological markers (CT and CEA) must be assessed; their stability advocating therapeutic abstention.

Prognosis

The MTC prognosis is essentially related to the anatomoclinic stage : Biological cure (normal CT) is achieved in almost all patients with no lymph node metastasis, while only 33-50% of patients are biologically cured when there is lymph node involvement [42, 59].When the disease is localized to the thyroid gland, the 10-year survival rate reaches 95.6% [37]. Patients with regional lymph node disease have a 5-year overall survival rate of 75.5%. Distant metastases are seen in 13% of patients at initial diagnosis, and these patients have a poor prognosis, with a 10-year survival rate of only 40% [37].

Conclusion

Systematic CT dosage for any thyroid nodule may allow early diagnosis of MTC. This will manifestly improve the prognosis of this disease which complete surgery remains the only curative treatment. In cases of distant or recurrent disease not amenable to surgery, there are promising new treatment options.

Screening of familial forms must be systematic in any MTC. The discovery of this hereditary forms requires specialized management.

References

[1] Saad MF, Ordonez NG, Rashid RK et al. Medullary carcinoma of the thyroid. A study of the clinical features and prognostic factors in 161 patients. *Medicine* (Baltimore) 1984;63:319 –342.

[2] Dottorini ME, Assi A, SironiMet al. Multivariate analysis of patients with medullary thyroid carcinoma. Prognostic significance and impact on treatment of clinical and pathologic variables. *Cancer* 1996;77:1556 –1565.

[3] Mure A, Gicquel C, Abdelmoumene N et al. Cushing's syndrome in medullary thyroid carcinoma. *J Endocrinol Invest* 1995;18:180 –185.

[4] Smallridge RC, Bourne K, Pearson BW et al. Cushing's syndrome due to medullary thyroid carcinoma: Diagnosis by proopiomelanocortin messenger ribonucleic acid in situ hybridization. *J Clin Endocrinol Metab* 2003;88:4565– 4568.

[5] Kloos RT, Eng C, Evans DB, Francis GL, Gagel RF, Gharib H, Moley JF, Pacini F, Ringel MD, Schlumberger M, Wells SA, Jr. Medullary thyroid cancer: management guidelines of the American Thyroid Association. *Thyroid* 2009;19: 565-612.

[6] Pacini F, Schlumberger M, Dralle H, Elisei R, Smit JW, Wiersinga W. European consensus for the management of patients with differentiated thyroid carcinoma of the follicular epithelium. *Eur J Endocrinol* 2006;154: 787-803.

[7] Elisei R, Bottici V, Luchetti F, et al. Impact of routine measurement of serum calcitonin on the diagnosis and outcome of medullary thyroid cancer: experience in 10 864 patients with nodular thyroid disorders. *J Clin Endocrinol Metab* 2004;89:163–8.

[8] Hahms JR, Lee MS, Min YK, et al. Routine measurement of serum calcitonin is useful for early detection of medullary thyroid carcinoma in patients with nodular thyroid diseases. *Thyroid* 2001;11:73–80.

[9] Karges W, Dralle H, Raue F, et al. Calcitonin measurement to detect medullary thyroid carcinoma in nodular goiter: german evidenced-based consensus recommendations. *Exp Clin Endocrinol Diabetes* 2004;112:52–8.

[10] Niccoli P, Wion-Barbot N, Caron P, et al. Interest of routine measurement of serum calcitonin (CT): study in a large series of thyroidectomized patients. *J Clin Endocrinol Metab* 1997;82:338–41.

[11] Costante G, Durante C, Francis Z, Schlumberger M, Filetti S. Determination of calcitonin levels in C-cell disease: clinical interest and potential pitfalls. *Nat Clin Pract Endocrinol Metab* 2009;5: 35-44.

[12] Boi F, Maurelli I, Pinna G, et al. Calcitonin measurement in wash-out fluid from fine needle aspiration of neck masses in patients with primary and metastatic medullary thyroid carcinoma. *J Clin Endocrinol Metab* 2007;92:2115-2118.

[13] Kudo T, Miyauchi A, Ito Y, et al. Diagnosis of medullary thyroid carcinoma by calcitonin measurement in fine-needle aspiration biopsy specimens. *Thyroid* 2007;17:635-638.

[14] D'Herbomez M, Leclerc L, Vantyghem MG, et al. Clinical evaluation of a new sensitive calcitonin assay: study of specificity. *Clin Chim Acta* 2001;311:149–55.

[15] Cohen R, Campos MJ, Salaun C, et al. Preoperative calcitonin levels are predictive of tumor size and cure in medullary thyroid carcinoma. *J Clin Endocrinol Metab* 2000;85:919–22.

[16] Albores-Saavedra J, Monforte H, Nadjik M, Morales AR. C-cell hyperplasia in thyroid tissue adjacent to follicular cell tumors. *Hum Pathol* 1988;19:795–9.

[17] Gibelin H, Esique D, Jones C, et al. Increased calcitonin level in thyroid nodules without medullary carcinoma. *Br J Surg* 2005;92:574–8.

[18] Karanikas G, Moameni A, Poetzi C, et al. Frequency and relevance of elevated calcitonin levels in patients with neoplasic and non-neoplasic thyroid disease and in healthy subjects. *J Clin Endocrinol Metab* 2004; 89:515–9.

[19] Niccoli P, Brunet P, Roubicek C, et al. Abnormal basal calcitonin level and pentagastrin response in patients with chronic renal failure on maintenance hemodialysis. *Eur J Endocrinol* 1995;132:75–81.

[20] Lissak B, Baudin E, Cohen R, et al. Pentagastrin testing in patients with renal insuficiency: normal responsivity of mature calcitonin. *Thyroid* 1998;8:265–8.

[21] Barbot N, Calmettes C, Schuffenecker I, et al. Pentagastrin stimulation test and early diagnosis of medullary carcinoma using an immunoradiometric assay of calcitonin: comparison with genetic screening in hereditary medullary thyroid carcinoma. *J Clin Endocrinol* Metab 1994;78:114–20.

[22] Wion-Barbot N, Schuffenecker I, Niccoli P, et al. Results of the calcitonin stimulation test in normal volunteers compared with genetically unaffected members of MEN 2A and familial medullary thyroid carcinoma families. *Ann Endocrinol* (Paris) 1997;58:302–8.

[23] Iacobone M, Niccoli-Sire P, Sebag F, et al. Can sporadic medullary thyroid carcinoma be biochemically predicted? Prospective analysis of 66 operated patients with elevated serum calcitonin levels. *World J Surg* 2002;26:886–90.

[24] Kaserer K, Scheuba C, Neuhold N, et al. C-cell hyperplasia and medullary thyroid carcinoma in patients routinely screened for serum calcitonin. *Am J Surg Pathol* 1998;22:722–8.

[25] Machens A, Dralle H. Pretargeted anti-carcinoembryonic-antigen radioimmunotherapy for medullary thyroid carcinoma. *J Clin Oncol* 2006;24:e37.

[26] Verga U, Fugazzola L, Cambiaghi S et al. Frequent association between MEN 2A and cutaneous lichen amyloidosis. *Clin Endocrinol* (Oxf) 2003;59:156–161.

[27] Moore SW, Zaahl M. Familial associations in medullary thyroid carcinoma with Hirschsprung disease:The role of the RET-C620 “Janus” genetic variation. *J Pediatr Surg* 2010;45:393–396.

[28] O’Riordain DS, O’Brien T, Crotty TB et al. Multiple endocrine neoplasia type 2B:Morethan an endocrine disorder. *Surgery* 1995;118:936 –942.

[29] Mulligan LM, Eng C, Healey CS et al. Specificmutations of the RET proto-oncogene are related to disease phenotype inMEN2A and FMTC. *Nat Genet* 1994;6:70 –74.

[30] Donis-Keller H, Dou S, Chi D et al. Mutations in the RET proto-oncogene are associated with MEN2A and FMTC. *Hum Mol Genet* 1993;2:851– 856.

[31] Brandi ML, Gagel RF, Angeli A et al. Guidelines for diagnosis and therapy of MEN type 1 and type 2. *J Clin Endocrinol Metab* 2001;86:5658 –5671.

[32] Niccoli-Sire P, Conte-Devolx B. Multiple endocrine neoplasia type 2: respective parts of biochemical and molecular genetic analysis in the diagnosis and management. *Immunoanalyse Biol Spécialisée* 2003;18:320–8.

[33] Niccoli-Sire P, Murat A, Rohmer V, et al. Familial medullary thyroid carcinoma (FMTC) with non-cysteine RET mutations: phenotype genotype relationship in a large series of patients. *J Clin Endocrinol* Metab 2001;86:3746–53.

[34] Ganeshan D, Paulson E, Duran C et al. Current Update on Medullary Thyroid Carcinoma. *AJR* 2013; 201: 867 – 876.

[35] Moley JF, DeBenedetti MK. Patterns of nodal metastases in palpable medullary thyroid carcinoma: Recommendations for extent of node dissection. *Ann Surg* 1999;229:880–887, discussion 887–888.

[36] Greenblatt DY, Elson D, Mack E et al. Initial lymph node dissection increases cure rates in patients with medullary thyroid cancer. *Asian J Surg* 2007;30:108 –112.

[37] Rebecca S. Sippel, Muthusamy Kunnimalaiyaan, Herbert Chen. Current Management of Medullary Thyroid Cancer. *The Oncologist* 2008;13:539–547.

[38] Machens A, Dralle H. Biomarker-based risk stratification for previously untreated medullary thyroid cancer. *J Clin Endocrinol Metab* 2010;95: 2655-2663.

[39] Machens A, Hauptmann S, Dralle H. Increased risk of lymph node metastasis in multifocal hereditary and sporadic medullary thyroid cancer. *World J Surg* 2007;31:1960 –1965.

[40] Scollo C, Baudin E, Travagli JP et al. Rationale for central and bilateral lymph node dissection in sporadic and hereditary medullary thyroid cancer. *J Clin Endocrinol Metab* 2003;88:2070 –2075.

[41] Machens A, Hinze R, Thomusch O, Dralle H. Pattern of nodal metastasis for primary and reoperative thyroid cancer. *World J Surg* 2002;28:22–8.

[42] Tamagnini P, Iacobone M, Sebag F, and al. Lymph node involvement in macroscopic medullary thyroid carcinoma. *Br J Surg* 2005;92:449–53.

[43] Leboulleux S, Travagli JP, Caillou B, Laplanche A, Bidart JM, Schlumberger M, Baudin E. Medullary thyroid carcinoma as part of a multiple endocrine neoplasia type 2B syndrome: influence of the stage on the clinical course. *Cancer* 2002;94: 44-50.

[44] Brauckhoff M, Machens A, Lorenz K, Bjoro T, Varhaug JE, Dralle H. Surgical Curability of Medullary Thyroid Cancer in Multiple Endocrine Neoplasia 2B: A Changing Perspective. *Ann Surg* 2013. Sep 20.

[45] Rohmer V, Vidal-Trecan G, Bourdelot A, Niccoli P, Murat A, Wemeau JL and al. Prognostic factors of disease-free survival after thyroidectomy in 170 young patients with a RET germline mutation: a multicenter study of the Groupe Francais d'Etude des Tumeurs Endocrines. *J Clin Endocrinol Metab* 2011;96: E509-518.

[46] Hyer SL, Vini L, A'Hern R, Harmer C. Medullary thyroid cancer: multivariate analysis of prognostic factors influencing survival. *Eur J Surg Oncol* 2000;26:686–90.

[47] Wilson PC, Millar BM, Brierley JD. The management of advanced thyroid cancer. *Clin Oncol* 2004;16:561–568.

[48] Nocera M, Baudin E, Pellegritti G, et al. Treatment of advanced medullary thyroid cancer with an alternating combination of doxorubicinstreptozotocin and 5 FU-dacarbazine. *Br J Cancer* 2000;83:715–8.

[49] Orlandi F, Caraci P, Berruti A, et al. Chemotherapy with dacarbazine and 5-Fluorouracil in advanced medullary thyroid cancer. *Ann Oncol* 1994;5:763–5.

[50] Stein R, Chen S, Reed L, et al. Combining radioimmunotherapy and chemotherapy for treatment of medullary thyroid carcinoma. *Effectiveness of Dacarbazine Cancer* 2002;94:51–61.

[51] Gild ML, Bullock M, Robinson BG, Clifton-Bligh R: Multikinase inhibitors: a new option for the treatment of thyroid cancer. *Nat Rev* Endocrinol 2011, 7(10):617-24.

[52] Kapiteijn E, Schneider TC, Morreau H, Gelderblom H, Nortier JW, Smit JW: New treatment modalities in advanced thyroid cancer. *Ann Oncol* 2012, 23(1):10-8.

[53] Pasieka JL, McEwan AJ, Rorstad O: The palliative role of 131 I-MIBG and 111 In-octreotide therapy in patients with metastatic progressive neuroendocrine neoplasms. *Surgery* 2004, 136:1218-1226.

[54] Kraeber-Bodere F, Goldenberg DM, Chatal JF, Barbet J: Pretargeted radioimmunotherapy in the treatment of metastatic medullary thyroid cancer. *Curr Oncol* 2009, 16:3-8.

[55] Brauckhoff M, Gimm O, Brauckhoff K, Ukkat J, Thomusch O, Dralle H. Calcitonin kinetics in the early postoperative period of medullary thyroid carcinoma. *Langenbecks Arch Surg* 2001;386(6): 434-439.

[56] Ismailov SI, Piulatova NR. Postoperative calcitonin study in medullary thyroid carcinoma. *Endocr Relat Cancer* 2004;11: 357-363.

[57] Machens A, Dralle H. Benefit-risk balance of reoperation for persistent medullary thyroid cancer. *Ann Surg* 2013;257: 751-757.

[58] Chen H, Roberts JR, BallDWet al. Effective long-term palliation of symptomatic, incurable metastatic medullary thyroid cancer by operative resection. *Ann Surg* 1998;227:887– 895.

[59] Machens A, Gimm O, Ukkat J, et al. Improved prediction of calcitonin normalisation in medullary thyroid carcinoma patients by quantitative lymph node analysis. *Cancer* 2000;88:1909–15.

In: Thyroid Nodules
Editor: Marsha Vasquez
ISBN: 978-1-63483-592-3

Chapter VI

Complications of Thyroidectomy: Risk Factors and Management

***Moncef Sellami**, *Souha Kallel*,
Mohamed Amine Chaabouni, *Ilhem Charfeddine*,
Boutheina Hammami and *Abdelmonem Ghorbel***
Department of otorhinolaryngology-Head and Neck Surgery
Habib Bourguiba University Hospital,
Sfax, Tunisia

Abstract

Thyroidectomy is a relatively common procedure and like any surgery procedure involves risks.

Thyroidectomy poses many challenges for the surgeon who undertakes endocrine surgery. Fatal complications are rare, but the incidence of minor complications and their sequelae are common.

The recurrent laryngeal nerve injury and hypocalcemia due to hypoparathyroidism are the most common early complications after a thyroid operation.

Hypocalcemia is generally transient, but it may be permanent requiring lifelong administration of calcium plus vitamin D.

* Phone : +21624050980. E-mail: sellami_moncef@yahoo.fr

Unilateral recurrent laryngeal nerve injury results in hoarseness or dysphonia due to laryngeal paralysis with unilateral vocal cord immobility. Bilateral recurrent laryngeal nerve palsy results in dramatic symptoms of acute life-threatening dyspnea.

Other complications of thyroid surgery include postoperative hemorrhage, seroma, hematoma, respiratory obstruction, wound infection and sepsis.

Risk factors of most complications should be considered before surgery.

In this chapter, we propose to study the complications of thyroidectomy as well as risk factors and current treatment modalities based on an evaluation of the recent studies of morbidity.

Introduction

Thyroidectomy is a common procedure with > 90,000 operations performed in the United States each year [1].

In this surgery, fatal complications are rare but the incidence of minor complications and their sequelae are common.

Today morbidity remains a subject of concern for surgeons performing thyroid surgery [2, 3]. Injury of the recurrent laryngeal nerve and hypoparathyroidism are the two classical complications specific to thyroidectomy due to the close anatomic proximity of the thyroid gland with the recurrent laryngeal nerves and parathyroid glands.

Other complications include superior laryngeal nerve injury, infection, airway compromise, and hematoma.

Postoperative compressive hematoma with acute dyspnea is a rare but severe complication that may result in death or severe long-term sequelae [4].

We propose to study specific and general complications of thyroidectomy as well as risk factors and current treatment modalities based on an evaluation of the recent studies of morbidity.

Specific Complications

Hypocalcemia

Hypocalcemia may be the only complication precluding a short postoperative hospital stay after total thyroidectomy.

The parathyroid glands, via the action of the parathyroid hormone (PTH), are responsible for maintaining of calcium homeostasis. Insufficient secretion or action of PTH manifests as hypocalcemia [2, 5].

Hypocalcemia after total thyroidectomy is common and its incidence varies from 2% to 83% [3]. In Table 1 we report some results of studies about postoperative hypothyroidism

Postsurgical hypocalcemia may be transient or permanent. Permanent hypocalcemia or hypoparathyroidism is defined by most studies as insufficient PTH to maintain normocalcemia 6 months after surgery [6, 7]. Transient hypoparathyroidism has been reported to occur significantly more often than permanent hypothyroidism following thyroid surgery, with an incidence ranging anywhere from 6.9% to 46% for the former, and from 0.9% to 1.6% for the latter [7].

Table 1. Incidence of post-operative transient and permanent hypocalcemia

Author	Number of patients	Year of publication	Transient Hypoclcemia	Permanent Hypocalcemia
Thomusch [8]	7266	2000	6,4%	1,5%
Efremidou EI [9]	932	2008	7,3%	0,3%
Abboud [4]	1127	2012	18%	0,8%
Seo ST [10]	349	2015	28%	13%
Ritter [11]	1054	2015	13%	1,9%

Risk Factors

Numerous studies have evaluated the risk of post-thyroidectomy hypoparathyroidism. The risk of postoperative hypocalcemia, whether transient or permanent, is increased by several factors:

Surgery-Related Factors

In a recent study [12] we found that parathyroid tissue present on pathology report was an independent risk factor for developing transient and permanent hypoparathyroidism. This result was in accordance with the literature [11]. A controversial debate exists about the number of parathyroid glands that should be identified and preserved during thyroid surgery in order to avoid postoperative hypocalcemia. Fewer parathyroid gland identified at operation is associated with transient and permanent hypocalcemia [2].

Severe reduction of visibility during diffuse bleeding from dissected thyroid tissue obviously leads more frequently to injuries of the parathyroid glands [8].

Local conditions can increase the risk of postoperative hypocalcemia such as large Grave's disease, goiter surgery, or thyroid cancer requiring nodal dissection often results in a removal of the lower parathyroid glands. Reoperation for recurrent goiter and concomitant central neck dissection for cancer thyroid may increase the risk of incidental parathyroidectomy [13]. This is due to the important postoperative fibrosis.

The complication rate is higher when the operation is done by inexperienced surgeon who have no special skills in endocrine surgery [14].

Biochemical Factors

Several studies demonstrated that the preoperative calcium level was significantly lower in patients who developed transient hypocalcemia. A preoperative calcium level of 2·27 mmol/l or lower had a good sensitivity for predicting transient hypocalcemia [15].

Intraoperative PTH level at any time after resection of the thyroid gland to 10 min after skin closure and lower postoperative PTH levels 30 min to 5 days after surgery are associated with transient hypocalcemia [16, 17].

A decline in PTH level from preoperative values to intraoperative levels measured 10–20 min after thyroid resection was also associated with transient hypocalcemia [16].

Recent studies found that pre-operative vitamin D status did not predict a postoperative decrease in serum calcium [18, 19]. Thus, routine preoperative screening for vitamin D is not recommended.

Symptoms

Symptoms of hypocalcemia most commonly include paresthesia, muscle spasms, cramps, tetany, and seizures. It can also present with laryngospasm, neuromuscular irritability, cognitive impairment, personality disturbances, prolonged QT intervals, electrocardiographic changes that mimic myocardial infarction, or heart failure [5].

The major risk of profound hypocalcemia is cardiac decompensation due to arrhythmias.

Biological Diagnosis

In the absence of any reliable predictors of clinically relevant hypocalcemia after total thyroidectomy, monitoring serum calcium concentrations has been considered the standard of care. Hypocalcemia typically presents within the first 2 days postoperatively [17].

Hypocalcemia is defined as a total serum calcium level less than 2 mM/L (8.0 mg/dL) or an ionized calcium level less than 1.1mM/L (0.275 mg/dL) [9].

Tartaglia et al. found higher correlations between ionized calcium concentrations and hypocalcemic symptoms, and recommend initiating treatment early, before patients develop acute hypocalcemia [20]. They concluded that ionized calcium is a more reliable parameter than total calcium in the immediate postoperative follow-up.

Treatment

A multidisciplinary approach is imperative to reduce the morbidity associated with hypoparathyroidism.

There is no consensus regarding the treatment of postoperative hypoparathyroidism. Measurement of calcium and PTH levels should ideally be performed six hours after the surgery [3, 17].

Acute symptomatic hypocalcemia requires treatment with IV calcium until ionized calcium levels are equal to or greater than 1.0 mmol/L [6].

Oral replacement of calcium, in addition to vitamin D supplementation should be initiated. Oral Calcium (dosing can range from 1 to 9 g per day) is usually given every 6 hours [7].

Vitamin D is administered as calcitriol at an initial dose of 0.5-1 μg twice a day. Doses should be adapted based on weekly measurement of calcium and phosphate levels until biological equilibrium is reached [3].

The protocol used at Monash University Endocrine Surgery Unit [21] is shown in Figure 1.

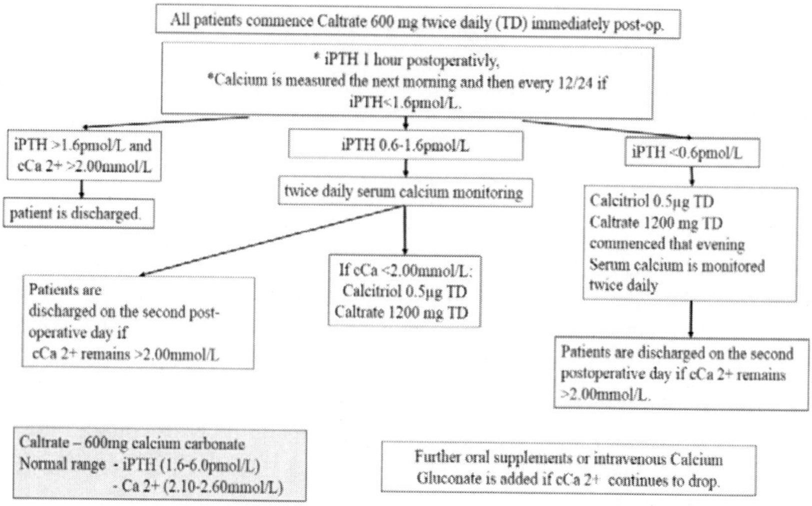

Figure 1. The Monash University Endocrine Surgery Unit postthyroidectomy calcium protocol (Caltrate = 600 mg calcium carbonate. Normal range: iPTH = 1.6–6.0 pmol/L; Ca 2+ = 2.10–2.60 mmol/L) [21].

Grodski et al. also proposed a discharge calcium protocol [21]:

- If patient is just on Caltrate tablets
    - On discharge they will normally be on: Caltrate 2 tablets, twice daily
    - If calcium is >2.00mmol/L at one week, reduce to: Caltrate 1 tablet, twice daily
    - If calcium is >2.00mmol/L the next week, reduce to: Caltrate 1 tablet daily
    - If calcium is normal the next week: Cease Caltrate
- If patient is on Caltrate + Rocaltrol (calcitriol) tablets:
    - On discharge they will normally be on: Caltrate 2 tablets, three times daily and Rocaltrol 2 tablets, twice daily
    - If calcium is >2.00mmol/L at one week, reduce to: Caltrate 2 twice daily and Rocaltrol 1 twice daily
    - If calcium is >2.00mmol/L the next week, reduce to: Caltrate 1 twice daily and Rocaltrol 1 daily
    - If calcium is >2.00mmol/L the next week, reduce to: Caltrate 1 daily
    - If calcium is normal the next week: Cease Caltrate

Prevention

Preservation of the parathyroid glands can be achieved during thyroidectomy, by systematic search for the parathyroid glands with visualization/sparing of at least two of them and careful protection of their vascular supply by meticulous dissection and sparing of the peri-glandular fat [22].

We prefer individual ligation of peripheral branches of the inferior thyroid artery rather than ligation of the main trunk to preserve the blood supply to the parathyroid glands during thyroid dissection. It has been reported that administration of post-thyroidectomy oral calcium with vitamin D did not appear to inhibit the function of normal parathyroid glands. A meta-analysis conducted by Alhefdhi et al. [23] found a significant decrease in the rate of symptomatic postoperative hypocalcemia between the groups treated with vitamin D along with calcium as compared to no prophylaxis or calcium alone. The results showed that the combination vitamin D with calcium is the most effective strategy. The author's recommendation regarding prophylactic calcium and/or vitamin D therapy for patients after thyroidectomy were:

- Postoperative oral calcium at a minimum dose of 3 g/day should be routinely given to all patients for 2 weeks following thyroid surgery.
- Patients who are at increased risk of postoperative hypocalcemia should be treated with the same calcium regimen, along with the addition of calcitriol at a dose of 1 µg/day.

When a prophylactic calcium/ vitamin D postoperative supplementation is prescribed treatment is ended within an average of 15 days after surgery, using progressively decreasing doses of calcitriol and calcium (lowered by 0.5 µg of calcitriol and 125 mg of calcium every 3 to 5 days), and monitoring total serum concentration of calcium at every change of dosage [24].

Recurrent Laryngeal Nerve Injury

Recurrent laryngeal nerve (RLN) injury is one of the most serious complications in endocrine surgery.

Transient post-operative recurrent laryngeal nerve palsy (RLNP) occurs in 1–8% of cases and permanent palsies in approximately 0.2–5% of cases [25] (Table 2). Bilateral palsy is exceptional.

Table 2. Incidence of transient and permanent recurrent laryngeal nerve palsy after thyroidectomy in large series

Author	Number of patients	Number of nerves at risk	Transient RLNP (%)		Permanent RLNP (%)	
			Unilateral	Bilateral	Unilateral	Bilateral
Chiang [26]	521	678	5,1%	0	5%	0
Abboud B [4]	1127	1927	5%	0	0,6%	0
Efremidou EI [9]	932	1864	1,3%	0	0,2%	0
Testini [27]	14993	29986	3,5%	0,2%	1,1%	0,002%

RLNP: recurrent laryngeal nerve palsy.

Risk Factors

Causes of nerve palsy include damage to the nerve's anatomic integrity, thermal lesions, excessive nerve skeletisation, axon damage caused by excessive strain, oedema, haematoma and difficult tracheal intubation and neuritis caused by scar tissue and viral neuritis [13]

There is a risk of recurrent nerve injury after any thyroid surgery.

Re-Operative Surgery

Thyroid reoperations can be challenging, even for a highly experienced thyroid surgeon, as visual identification of the RLN is more difficult during dissection of the tissues than in the virgin neck [28].

Cancer Surgery

Lymph node dissection increases the rates of complications. In a retrospective study of 186 dissected recurrent nerves, we found that the RLNP increased by the presence of cancer requiring a central nodal dissection [29].

Extent of Surgery

Erbil et al. in a retrospective study analyzing 3250 patients, reported a 12 fold increased risk of RLNP in patients undergoing extended thyroidectomy (lobectomy or total thyroidectomy) compared with conservative surgery (subtotal resection) [13].

Thyroid Pathology

- Graves' disease:

The presence of chronic thyroiditis or Grave's disease increase the risk of recurrent nerve injury [30].

- Retrosternal goiter:

During surgery of retrosternal goiter, the nerve is stretched and more exposed to injury. Testini [27] found that the extension of the goiter into the mediastinum (50 among 14,993 total thyroidectomies) was associated to increased risk of recurrent nerve palsy.

Surgeon Experience

In many studies, the experience of the surgeon has been found to be a significant factor related to the incidence of complications following thyroid surgery.

Dralle et al. defined surgical experience with regard to RLN treatment that was given by the number of nerves at risk NAR , surgeon volume was categorized according to the total volume of operated sites (NAR) per year: surgeons with <45 vs ≥ 45 operated thyroid sites. The authors reported RLNP rates of 0.72% for surgeons performing greater than 45 NAR procedures per year compared with 1.06% in those with less than 45 NAR per year (p= 0.003), with both groups having similar surgery types and pathology [30].

Clinical Presentation

Damage to a recurrent laryngeal nerve with resultant paralysis of the sole abducting muscle (posterior cricoarytenoid) of the vocal cords can cause symptoms ranging from almost undetectable hoarseness in unilateral lesions to stridor and acute airway obstruction in bilateral injury.

Unilateral recurrent laryngeal nerve injury results in hoarseness or dysphonia due to laryngeal paralysis with unilateral vocal cord immobility and is often associated with upper airway dyspnea and swallowing problems [3].

The rare bilateral recurrent laryngeal nerve palsy results in dramatic symptoms of acute life-threatening dyspnea or serious swallowing problems [3].

Diagnosis

Indirect mirror laryngoscopy or fiberoptic laryngoscopy performed postoperatively to evaluate the vocal folds function. Most laryngologists agree that flexible rather than rigid laryngoscopy provides the most accurate assessment of vocal fold mobility and degree of glottic insufficiency [31].

Vocal cord dysfunction is defined as [27]:

- paresis : hypomotility without paramedian paralysis
- paralysis: absence of motility and paramedian position.

Videostroboscopy provides further information on associated vocal fold vibratory perturbations and also provides a complete evaluation of vocal fold closure [32].

Treatment

Unilateral Recurrent Nerve Injury

If a unilateral recurrent nerve injury is well tolerated (paralyzed vocal cord stays in the paramedian position), simple surveillance should continue for at least six months before intervention since spontaneous recovery of nerve function is possible [33].

Severe respiratory difficulties, pneumonia and poor vocal quality should be the indications for surgery [34].

Most practitioners accept that a waiting time between 6 and 12 months is appropriate before considering framework surgery [34, 35].

An optimal glottal closure ,as well as symmetrical vocal fold masses, and tensions are essential prerequisites for normal voice production. Successful phonosurgery depends on restoring these prerequisites to achieve long-term improvement. Several remedial surgical techniques have been proposed :

- Medialization thyroplasty:

Through a short horizontal incision in the neck, a window is drilled in the cartilage of the thyroid ala for insertion of an implant into the paralyzed vocal cord. Implant materials are divided into autologous and synthetic. Autologous implant materials include fat, fascia, muscle, and cartilage. These materials are not widely used due to the unpredictable nature of their long-term medialization related to variable absorption and migration. Synthetic materials include Silastic®, Gore-Tex®, and others [32].

- Intracordal injection:

Medialization of the vocal cord by intracordal injection of autologous material (fat) or heterologous material (silicone, collagen) via endoscopic or trans-cutaneous route [3]. Autologous fat does not disturb vocal cord vibration, even when injected into the superficial layer of the lamina propria and is superior to other materials for vocal rehabilitation [36].

- Arytenoid Adduction:

Adduction of the arytenoid muscle by placement of a traction suture. In most cases, the approach to the muscular process of arytenoid is accomplished through the same operative exposure used for implant placement [32].

Voice re-education is often prescribed; although it contributes nothing to reinnervation, it does result in improved respiratory function and also in a notable psychologic patient benefit [3]. Voice therapy can help inadequate breath support that can impair the post-operatively recovery process and confound functional voice outcomes [32].

In most of the cases, accidental injury to the recurrent laryngeal nerve is not recognized during surgery. If the surgeon is aware of this complication intraoperatively, primarily repair of the nerve using microsurgical techniques and epineural sutures or a nerve graft can be attempted. Even if the nerve is reanastomosed, the dysfunctioning vocal cord will probably never completely recover [33].

Bilateral Recurrent Nerve Injury

Bilateral nerve palsy is directly diagnosed after extubation or during the early postoperative phase. The patient should be reintubated without delay and treated systemically with corticosteroids. In the presence of reversible nerve injury, extubation under controlled conditions is done in most cases after 24–72 hours and no further treatment is necessary [33].

High-dose corticosteroid protocol is administered for 48 hours to decrease laryngeal edema (IV solumedrol 20 to 60 mg by slow IV infusion over 30 minutes every 8-12 hours, or dexamethasone 4 to 10 mg/day) [3].

In case of persisting respiratory obstruction (persistent vocal cord immobility and severe dyspnea) tracheostomy is often done but is not acceptable by patients as a long-term solution [37].

For patients showing no spontaneous functional recovery, several surgical techniques to achieve a glottis space enlargement are performed. We wait between 6 and 12 months, following the vocal cord palsy, before taking them up for definitive surgery.

The extralaryngeal approaches (ventriculocordectomy, submucosal vocal cord resection, laterofixation of the vocal cord and external arytenoidectomy) are replaced with less invasive endoscopic approaches including arytenoidectomy and posterior cordotomy [38, 39].

The posterior cordotomy technique of Dennis and Kashima using carbon dioxide laser posterior cordectomy consists of creation of a wedge-shaped opening in both the true and false vocal cord by retracting the thyroarytenoid muscle. It is a simple surgery, which leads to a predictable enlargement of the glottic space while preserving good final voice quality and swallowing functions [39].

The total arytenoidectomy described by Ossoff et al. [38] leads to the formation of granulation tissue and scarring, which may further obstruct the lumen.

Danino et al. proposed the use of the submucosal approach, to excise the arytenoid cartilage. Submucosal approach was associated with good resulting airway, minimal compromise of phonation and prevent granulation [40].

Remacle et al. described a subtotal carbon dioxide (CO2) laser arytenoidectomy which is a variant of total arytenoidectomy [41].

Combining posterior partial cordotomy as described by Dennis and Kashima [39], with total arytenoidectomy as described by Ossoff et al. [38] provides significant and stable improvement of respiratory function and, decrease the chance of reoperation with acceptable voice quality and no degree of aspiration [42].

Prevention

Prevention of laryngeal nerve injury depends on meticulously careful dissection and visualization of the nerves.

The thyroid surgeon must be aware of the possible anatomical variations of the nerve (figure 2), and always search for its visual control and gentle dissection, which are imperative since possible mechanisms of injury include transection, clamping, ligation, traction, thermal injury, and ischemia [43].

Intraoperative identification and capsular dissection are crucial in the preservation of the RLN [25, 30].

Intraoperative neural monitoring (IONM) during thyroid surgery has gained widespread acceptance as an adjunct to the gold standard of visual nerve identification [44].

A meta-analysis, which included twenty studies comparing thyroidectomy with and without intraoperative nerve monitoring (IONM), showed no statistically significant difference in the incidence of RLN palsy when using IONM versus visualization alone during thyroidectomy [44].

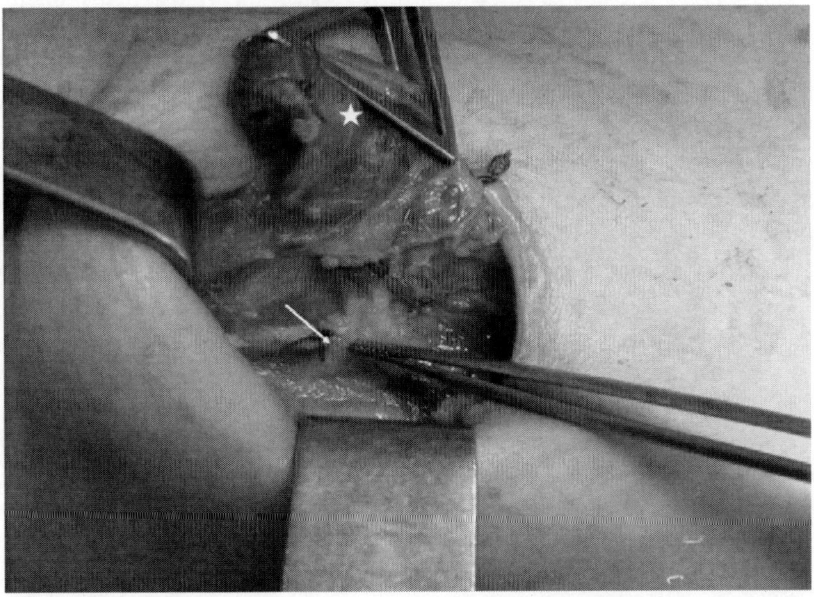

Figure 2. A non-recurrent inferior laryngeal nerve on the right side: the thyroid lobe is reclined (star) and the nerve (arrow) runs horizontally from the vagus toward the larynx.

External Branch of the Superior Laryngeal Nerve Injury

Injury of the external branch of the superior laryngeal nerve (EBSLN) during thyroid surgery can occur during the dissection and ligation of the superior thyroid vessels in up to 58% of patients.

The EBSLN paralysis results in dysfunction of the cricothyroid muscle, which results in altered fundamental frequency of the voice, a deterioration in voice performance in producing high-frequency sounds, and reduced vocal projection [43]. The clinical signs of EBSLN injury include hoarseness, decreased voice projection, decreased pitch range, and fatigue after extensive voice use [45]. This can have catastrophic consequences in people who use their voice professionally [46]. Fiberoptic laryngoscopy shows a remarkably normal motility of the vocal cords [43]. The diagnosis is made by videostroboscopy (which evaluates the regularity and symmetry of the mucosal traveling wave and the degree of glottis closure) and/or electromyography of the cricothyroid (that documents a decreased recruitment, and polyphasic action potentials that might reach the electrical silence in extreme cases) [43].

Care must be taken to avoid both the stretching of the nerve and an indiscriminate use of monopolar diathermy or energy-based devices for sealing vessels, in order to prevent iatrogenic heat injuries [43].

The EBSLN may not be able to be visualized in up to 20% of cases and the International Neural Monitoring Study Group Standards Guideline Statement recommend using the IONM to identify the EBSLN [46]. The use of the IONM improves the identification rate of the EBSLN during surgery to reduce voice impairment [47].

No surgical treatment is required after EBSLN injury; the management consists of voice re-education and administration of aerosolized corticosteroids [3].

Nonspecific Complications

Postoperative Hematoma

The thyroid is a highly vascularized organ which blood flow exceeds that of other highly perfused organs, such as the brain [48]. Although uncommon, postoperative hematoma is a potentially life-threatening complication of thyroid surgery.

The incidence of post-operative hematoma after surgery has been found to range from 0.2 to 4 percent [4].

Hematomas can result from inadequate hemostasis at the time of closure or increased venous pressure at the time of extubation because of coughing or straining [4].

Risk Factors

Postoperative hemorrhage has been attributed to three categories of risk [48, 49]:

- Surgical technique: use of a drain, extent of surgery, total thyroidectomy, which doubled the risk compared with a unilateral procedure.
- Patient predisposition: older age, male gender, active smoking, actively using antiplatelet, anticoagulation medication, previous thyroid operation and elevated postoperative blood pressure
- thyroid pathology: Graves' disease (increase the vascularity of the thyroid), large goiter, increased mass of the excised gland, the size of the dominant nodule, malignant histology,

Clinical Presentation

Cervical hematoma after thyroidectomy typically occurs within 24 h of surgery, with most significant hematomas becoming apparent within 6 to 8 h postoperatively [48, 50].

The diagnosis of wound hematoma is made by observing the neck and noticing a progressive collection under the skin or airway symptoms (Figure 3).

The extensive hematoma may produce respiratory failure and early intervention becomes necessary.

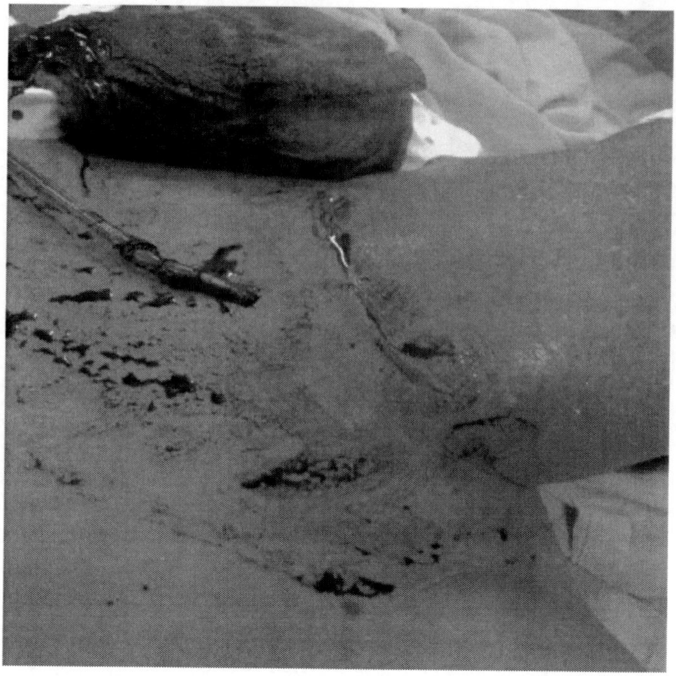

Figure 3. Postoperative cervical hematoma before surgical re-intervention (note the drain blocked by clots).

Treatment

In the event of hematoma formation, early surgical re-intervention is strongly advocated with due care given to at risk structures [51].

Re-intervention is strongly required in case of rapid accumulation of blood, with more than 150 ml in the suction bottle; visible swelling of the neck; or symptoms of airway compression [48].Surgical re-intervention clamping of vessels within the hematoma is to be avoided, and it is suggest to use of water to assist in identification of any bleeding points. The sources of the bleeding must be found and closed (ligation or coagulation). Suction drains are routinely employed at the end of exploration [51].

Patients with minimal swelling, absence of symptoms and no progression of hematoma should be considered for conservative management.

A minor hematoma might be detected within 2 weeks after discharge from hospital in the study of Abboud et al. [4]. The authors reported that some patients with seroma needed repeated aspirations.

Prevention

A meticulous hemostasis is more important than the use of drains, as neither drains nor bulky pressure dressings prevent hematoma development. In cases of major postoperative bleeding, drains are rapidly blocked by clots [4].

The use of drains post-thyroid surgery is systematic for all the surgeons [4, 48].

In a Cochrane revue entitled "Wound drains following thyroid surgery" [52] there was no clear evidence that using drains in patients undergoing thyroid operations significantly improves patient outcomes and drains may be associated with an increased length of hospital stay.

In our experience, we generally use a drain for 48 hours especially for:

- Resection of a substernal goiter and large goiter
- Older age
- Patients using antiplatelet or anticoagulation medication or patients
- Patients with previous thyroid operation
- Cases of hypervascularity, such as Grave disease or extensive cancers dissection.
- High blood pressure

Many surgeons believe that the use of a drain do not prevent a postoperative hematoma but allows better monitoring of the postoperative course in case of postoperative hematoma [27].

Wound Infection

Routine antibiotic prophylaxis is not recommended for clean surgical cases, and thyroidectomy is almost always classified as a clean case [53].

Rates of surgical site infections in thyroidectomy are quite low, reported to be between 0.3% and 3% in most series, but the consequences can be costly and morbid for patients [54].

In retrospective analysis, which included a total of 49326 patients underwent thyroidectomy, Elfenbein et al. reported that wound infection was independently associated with higher rates of wound dehiscence (OR 24.1, 95% CI,8.1-71.3), renal insufficiency (OR 70.4, 95% CI, 6.6-747.9), and acute renal failure (OR 35.7, 95% CI, 3.4-376.3), sepsis (OR 75.3, 95% CI, 35.1-161.5), and return to the operating room (OR 5.5, 95% CI, 3.5-8.9) [54]. Elfenbein et al. also found that patients who are obese, patients who are heavy users of alcohol, or those who are non-independent functional status should be considered higher risk for surgical site infections. These are the patients who may benefit most from selective use of antibiotic prophylaxis.

Minor cellulitis usually responds well to oral antibiotics directed at Staphylococcus and Streptococcus species [55]. Clinically evident seromas respond well to percutaneous aspiration [33].

Frank abscesses should be treated with incision and drainage. A delay of invasive treatment can result in devastating mediastinitis [33].

Lu Q et al. [56] suggest that the preventative use of antibacterials may not be required if the operation is performed under strict conditions of sterility and hemostasis and should only be considered if:

- the patient needs to take antibacterial medication for prevention or treatment of a basic condition, such as an infection diagnosed before surgery, serious/complicated heart/pulmonary conditions, and diabetes.
- the operation time exceeds 3 hours or bleeding exceeds more than 1500µmL
- additional neck lymph node resection is required for a malignant thyroid tumor.

Other Complications

Lymphorrhea

Lymphorrhea or chyle leak is an extremely rare complication of thyroidectomy and should be considered in the differential diagnosis of neck swelling postoperatively [57].

Chyle leak develops following central neck dissection as a result of injury to either the ascending part of the thoracic duct medial to the carotid sheath or, in some individuals, the duct terminating in the subclavian vein medial to the internal jugular vein [58].

Different management approaches were described:

- conservative approach consists of suction drains, compressive dressings, rest, and low fat diet (that is directly absorbed into the portal circulation resulting in reduced lymphatic flow of chylous fluid) or total parenteral nutrition [57, 59].
- surgical approach, by ligation of the thoracic duct, fibrin glue, or muscle flap, is reserved for patients who do not respond to conservative management (persistent drainage output >600 ml/day for 5–7 days) and for high output leakage (>1.5–2 L/day) [59].

Tracheal Injury

Tracheal injury following thyroidectomy is rare. In a review of 11917 patients over a 45-year period, Gosnell et al. identified seven patients with perforations for an incidence of 0.06% [60].

Risk factors for injury include female gender, thyrotoxic goiter, prolonged intubation with high cuff pressure, use of diathermy and persistent uncontrolled cough in the postoperative period [61, 62, 63]. The trachea may be perforated or lacerated intraoperatively, which is often recognized and repaired immediately with little patient morbidity [63]. However, unrecognized injury, or delayed rupture secondary to tracheal necrosis, can present up to 2 weeks postoperatively [61].

Thyrotoxic Storm

The thyrotoxic storm has largely disappeared since preoperative preparation with beta blockade and anti-thyroid medication has become routine practice [3]. The symptoms that may be seen are tachycardia, fever, nausea and vomiting, restlessness, mental stimulation, and frequently coma [33].

Mortality after Thyroid Surgery

Thyroidectomy is considered to be a safe procedure. Although very uncommon, death may occur after thyroid resection.

Mortality after thyroidectomy approaches 0%.

In a study of 30.495 thyroidectomies, postoperative mortality was 0,065% and its causes were [50]:

- Hematoma (0%)
- Respiratory distress/pneumonia due to prolonged endotracheal intubation (25%)
- Tracheal injury (15%)
- Heart failure (15%),
- Sepsis (wound infection/esophageal perforation) (10%)
- Mycotic aneurysm (5%).

Conclusion

Thyroidectomy is a safe procedure often performed either for benign or malignant thyroid diseases. Most complications of thyroid surgery are related to either metabolic derangements or injury to the recurrent laryngeal nerves.

There should be a systematic strategy for detection of complications after thyroidectomy involving a multidisciplinary approach.

References

[1] Sun GH, DeMonner S, Davis MM. Epidemiological and economic trends in inpatient and outpatient thyroidectomy in the United States, 1996-2006. *Thyroid.* 2013 Jun;23(6):727-33.

[2] Bergenfelz A, Jansson S, Kristoffersson A, Mårtensson H, Reihnér E, Wallin G, Lausen I. Complications to thyroid surgery: results as reported in a database from a multicenter audit comprising 3,660 patients. *Langenbecks Arch Surg*. 2008 Sep;393(5):667-73.

[3] Christou N, Mathonnet M. Complications after total thyroidectomy. J Visc Surg. 2013 Sep;150(4):249-56. doi: 10.1016/j.jviscsurg.2013.04.003. Epub 2013 Jun 6.

[4] Abboud B, Sleilaty G, Rizk H, Abadjian G, Ghorra C. Safety of thyroidectomy and cervical neck dissection without drains. *Can J Surg*. 2012 Jun;55(3):199-203.

[5] Al-Azem H, Khan AA. Hypocalcemia: updates in diagnosis and management for primary care. *Best Pract Res Clin Endocrinol Metab*. 2012 Aug;26(4):517-22.

[6] Walker Harris V, Jan De Beur S. Postoperative hypoparathyroidism: medical and surgical therapeutic options. *Thyroid*. 2009 Sep;19(9):967-73.

[7] Bilezikian JP, Khan A, Potts JT Jr, Brandi ML, Clarke BL, Shoback D, Jüppner H, D'Amour P, Fox J, Rejnmark L, Mosekilde L, Rubin MR, Dempster D, Gafni R, Collins MT, Sliney J, Sanders J. Hypoparathyroidism in the adult: epidemiology, diagnosis, pathophysiology, target-organ involvement, treatment, and challenges for future research. *J Bone Miner Res*. 2011 Oct;26(10):2317-37.

[8] Thomusch O, Machens A, Sekulla C, Ukkat J, Lippert H, Gastinger I, Dralle H. Multivariate analysis of risk factors for postoperative complications in benign goiter surgery: prospective multicenter study in Germany. *World J Surg*. 2000 Nov;24(11):1335-41.

[9] Efremidou EI, Papageorgiou MS, Liratzopoulos N, Manolas KJ. The efficacy and safety of total thyroidectomy in the management of benign thyroid disease: a review of 932 cases. *Can J Surg*. 2009 Feb;52(1):39-44.

[10] Seo ST, Chang JW, Jin J, Lim YC, Rha KS, Koo BS. Transient and permanent hypocalcemia after total thyroidectomy: Early predictive factors and long-term follow-up results. *Surgery*. 2015 Jul 2. pii: S0039-6060(15)00444-4.

[11] Ritter K, Elfenbein D, Schneider DF, Chen H, Sippel RS. Hypoparathyroidism after total thyroidectomy: incidence and resolution. *J Surg Res*. 2015 Aug;197(2):348-53.

[12] Sellami M, Achour I, Ben Said A, Kessentini A, Charfeddine I, Ghorbel A. La thyroïdectomie totale : étude de la morbidité spécifique. Annales françaises d'Oto-rhino-laryngologie et de Pathologie Cervico-faciale, Volume 131, Issue 4, Supplement, October 2014, Page A14.

[13] Erbil Y, Barbaros U, Işsever H, Borucu I, Salmaslioğlu A, Mete O, Bozbora A, Ozarmağan S. Predictive factors for recurrent laryngeal

nerve palsy and hypoparathyroidism after thyroid surgery. *Clin Otolaryngol.* 2007 Feb;32(1):32-7.

[14] Kotan C, Kösem M, Algün E, Ayakta H, Sönmez R, Söylemez O. Influence of the refinement of surgical technique and surgeon's experience on the rate of complications after total thyroidectomy for benign thyroid disease. *Acta Chir Belg*. 2003 Jun;103(3):278-81.

[15] Amir A, Sands NB, Tamilia M, Hier MP, Black MJ, Payne RJ. Preoperative serum calcium levels as an indicator of postthyroidectomy hypocalcemia. *J Otolaryngol Head Neck Surg*. 2010 Dec;39(6):654-8.

[16] Edafe O, Antakia R, Laskar N, Uttley L, Balasubramanian SP. Systematic review and meta-analysis of predictors of post-thyroidectomy hypocalcaemia. *Br J Surg*. 2014 Mar;101(4):307-20.

[17] Lecerf P, Orry D, Perrodeau E, Lhommet C, Charretier C, Mor C, Valat C, Bourlier P, de Calan L. Parathyroid hormone decline 4 hours after total thyroidectomy accurately predicts hypocalcemia. *Surgery.* 2012 Nov;152(5):863-8.

[18] Falcone TE, Stein DJ, Jumaily JS, Pearce EN, Holick MF, McAneny DB, Jalisi S, Grillone GA, Stone MD, Devaiah AK, Noordzij JP. Correlating pre-operative vitamin d status with post-thyroidectomy hypocalcemia. *Endocr Pract*. 2015 Apr 2;21(4):348-54.

[19] Lee GH, Ku YH, Kim HI, Lee MC, Kim MJ. Vitamin D level is not a predictor of hypocalcemia after total thyroidectomy. *Langenbecks Arch Surg.* 2015 Jun 9.

[20] Tartaglia F, Giuliani A, Sgueglia M, Patrizi G, Di Rocco G, Blasi S, Russo G, Tortorelli G, Giannotti D, Redler A. Is ionized calcium a reliable predictor of hypocalcemia after total thyroidectomy? A before and after study. *G Chir*. 2014 Jan-Feb;35(1-2):27-35.

[21] Grodski S, Serpell J. Evidence for the role of perioperative PTH measurement after total thyroidectomy as a predictor of hypocalcemia. *World J Surg*. 2008 Jul;32(7):1367-73.

[22] Giles Y1, Boztepe H, Terzioglu T, Tezelman S. The advantage of total thyroidectomy to avoid reoperation for incidental thyroid cancer in multinodular goiter. *Arch Surg.* 2004 Feb;139(2):179-82.

[23] Alhefdhi A, Mazeh H, Chen H. Role of postoperative vitamin D and/or calcium routine supplementation in preventing hypocalcemia after thyroidectomy: a systematic review and meta-analysis. *Oncologist.* 2013;18(5):533-42.

[24] Tartaglia F, Giuliani A, Sgueglia M, Biancari F, Juvonen T, Campana FP. Randomized study on oral administration of calcitriol to prevent

symptomatic hypocalcemia after total thyroidectomy. *Am J Surg*. 2005 Sep;190(3):424-9.

[25] Hayward NJ, Grodski S, Yeung M, Johnson WR, Serpell J. Recurrent laryngeal nerve injury in thyroid surgery: a review. *ANZ J Surg*. 2013 Jan;83(1-2):15-21. doi: 10.1111/j.1445-2197.2012.06247.x. Epub 2012 Sep 18.

[26] Feng-Yu Chiang, MD, Ling-Feng Wang, MD, Yin-Feng Huang, MD, Ka-Wo Lee, MD,. Recurrent laryngeal nerve palsy after thyroidectomy with routine identification of the recurrent laryngeal nerve.

[27] Testini M, Gurrado A, Bellantone R, Brazzarola P, Cortese R, De Toma G, Fabiola Franco I, Lissidini G, Pio Lombardi C, Minerva F, Di Meo G, Pasculli A, Piccinni G, Rosato L. Recurrent laryngeal nerve palsy and substernal goiter. An Italian multicenter study. *J Visc Surg*. 2014 Jun;151(3):183-9.

[28] Barczyński M1, Konturek A, Pragacz K, Papier A, Stopa M, Nowak W. Intraoperative nerve monitoring can reduce prevalence of recurrent laryngeal nerve injury in thyroid reoperations: results of a retrospective cohort study. *World J Surg*. 2014 Mar;38(3):599-606.

[29] Sellami M, Kallel S, Kessentini A, Ben Said A, Charfeddine I, Ghorbel A. Morbidité de l'évidement du compartiment central dans la chirurgie thyroïdienne. Annales françaises d'Oto-rhino-laryngologie et de Pathologie Cervico-faciale, Volume 131, Issue 4, Supplement, October 2014, Page A16.

[30] Dralle H, Sekulla C, Haerting J, Timmermann W, Neumann HJ, Kruse E, Grond S, Mühlig HP, Richter C, Voss J, Thomusch O, Lippert H, Gastinger I, Brauckhoff M, Gimm O. Risk factors of paralysis and functional outcome after recurrent laryngeal nerve monitoring in thyroid surgery. *Surgery*. 2004 Dec;136(6):1310-22.

[31] Fleischer S, Schade G, Hess MM. Office-based laryngoscopic observations of recurrent laryngeal nerve paresis and paralysis. . . *Ann Otol Rhinol Laryngol*. 2005;114:488–493.

[32] Daniero JJ, Garrett CG, Francis DO. Framework Surgery for Treatment of Unilateral Vocal Fold Paralysis. *Curr Otorhinolaryngol Rep*. 2014 Jun 1;2(2):119-130.

[33] Frilling A, Weber F (2007). Complications in Thyroid and Parathyroid Surgery. In: Oertli D, Udelsman R (eds) Surgery of the Thyroid and Parathyroid Glands. Springer, Philadelphia, PA, pp 217-223.

[34] Hartl DM, Travagli JP, Leboulleux S, Baudin E, Brasnu DF, Schlumberger M. Clinical review: Current concepts in the management

of unilateral recurrent laryngeal nerve paralysis after thyroid surgery. J *Clin Endocrinol Metab.* 2005 May;90(5):3084-8.

[35] Sulica L. The natural history of idiopathic unilateral vocal fold paralysis: evidence and problems. *Laryngoscope.* 2008;118:1303–1307.

[36] Tamura E, Fukuda H, Tabata Y. Intracordal injection technique: materials and injection site. *Tokai J Exp Clin Med.* 2008 Sep 20;33(3):119-23.

[37] Dispenza F, Dispenza C, Marchese D, Kulamarva G, Saraniti C. Treatment of bilateral vocal cord paralysis following permanent recurrent laryngeal nerve injury. *Am J Otolaryngol.* 2012 May-Jun;33(3):285-8.

[38] Ossoff RH, Sisson GA, Duncavage JA, Moselle HI, Andrews PE, McMillan WG. Endoscopic laser arytenoidectomy for the treatment of bilateral vocal cord paralysis. *Laryngoscope.* 1984 Oct;94(10):1293-7.

[39] Dennis DP, Kashima H. Carbon dioxide laser posterior cordectomy for treatment of bilateral vocal cord paralysis. *Ann Otol Rhinol Laryngol.* 1989 Dec;98(12 Pt 1):930-4.

[40] Danino J, Goldenberg D, Joachims HZ. Submucosal arytenoidectomy: new surgical technique and review of the literature. *J Otolaryngol.* 2000 Feb;29(1):13-6.

[41] Remacle M, Lawson G, Mayné A, Jamart J. Subtotal carbon dioxide laser arytenoidectomy by endoscopic approach for treatment of bilateral cord immobility in adduction. *Ann Otol Rhinol Laryngol.* 1996 Jun;105(6):438-45.

[42] Bizakis JG1, Papadakis CE, Karatzanis AD, Skoulakis CE, Kyrmizakis DE, Hajiioannou JK, Helidonis ES. The combined endoscopic CO(2) laser posterior cordectomy and total arytenoidectomy for treatment of bilateral vocal cord paralysis. *Clin Otolaryngol Allied Sci.* 2004 Feb;29(1):51-4.

[43] Varaldo E, Ansaldo GL, Mascherini M, Cafiero F1, Minuto MN1. Neurological complications in thyroid surgery: a surgical point of view on laryngeal nerves. *Front Endocrinol* (Lausanne). 2014 Jul 15;5:108.

[44] Pisanu A, Porceddu G, Podda M, Cois A, Uccheddu A. Systematic review with meta-analysis of studies comparing intraoperative neuromonitoring of recurrent laryngeal nerves versus visualization alone during thyroidectomy. *J Surg Res.* 2014 May 1;188(1):152-61.

[45] Kochilas X, Bibas A, Xenellis J, Anagnostopoulou S. Surgical anatomy of the external branch of the superior laryngeal nerve and its clinical

significance in head and neck surgery. *Clin Anat.* 2008 Mar;21(2):99-105.

[46] Barczyński M, Randolph GW, Cernea CR, Dralle H, Dionigi G, Alesina PF, Mihai R, Finck C, Lombardi D, Hartl DM, Miyauchi A, Serpell J, Snyder S, Volpi E, Woodson G, Kraimps JL, Hisham AN et Group., International Neural Monitoring Study. External branch of the superior laryngeal nerve monitoring during thyroid and parathyroid surgery: International Neural Monitoring Study Group standards guideline statement. *Laryngoscope.* 2013 Sep;123 Suppl 4:S1-14.

[47] Masuoka H, Miyauchi A, Higashiyama T, Yabuta T, Fukushima M, Ito Y, Kihara M, Kobayashi K, Yamada O, Nakayama A, Miya A. Prospective randomized study on injury of the external branch of the superior laryngeal nerve during thyroidectomy comparing intraoperative nerve monitoring and a conventional technique. *Head Neck.* 2014 May 21. doi: 10.1002/hed.23778. [Epub ahead of print].

[48] Promberger R, Ott J, Kober F, Koppitsch C, Seemann R, Freissmuth M, Hermann M. Risk factors for postoperative bleeding after thyroid surgery. *Br J Surg.* 2012 Mar;99(3):373-9.

[49] Campbell MJ, McCoy KL, Shen WT, Carty SE, Lubitz CC, Moalem J, Nehs M, Holm T,et al. A multi-institutional international study of risk factors for hematoma after thyroidectomy. *Surgery.* 2013 Dec;154(6):1283-89; discussion 1289-91.

[50] Gómez-Ramírez J, Sitges-Serra A, Moreno-Llorente P, Zambudio AR, Ortega-Serrano J, Rodríguez MT, Del Moral JV. Mortality after thyroid surgery, insignificant or still an issue? *Langenbecks Arch Surg.* 2015 May;400(4):517-22.

[51] Harding J, Sebag F, Sierra M, Palazzo FF, Henry JF. Thyroid surgery: postoperative hematoma--prevention and treatment. *Langenbecks Arch Surg.* 2006 Jun;391(3):169-73.

[52] Samraj K, Gurusamy KS. Wound drains following thyroid surgery. *Cochrane Database Syst Rev.* 2007 Oct 17;(4):CD006099.

[53] Mangram AJ, Horan TC, Pearson ML, Silver LC, Jarvis WR. Guideline for Prevention of Surgical Site Infection, 1999. Centers for Disease Control and Prevention (CDC) Hospital Infection Control Practices Advisory Committee. *Am J Infect Control.* 1999 Apr;27(2):97-132.

[54] Elfenbein DM, Schneider DF, Chen H, Sippel RS. Surgical site infection after thyroidectomy: a rare but significant complication. *J Surg Res.* 2014 Jul;190(1):170-6.

[55] Fewins J, Simpson CB, Miller FR. Complications of thyroid and parathyroid surgery. *Otolaryngol Clin North Am.* 2003 Feb;36(1):189-206, x.

[56] Lu Q, Xie SQ, Chen SY, Chen LJ, Qin Q. Experience of 1166 thyroidectomy without use of prophylactic antibiotic. *Biomed Res Int.* 2014;2014:758432.

[57] Rammal A, Zawawi F, Varshney R, Hier MP, Payne RJ, Mlynarek AM. Chyle leak: a rare complication post-hemithyroidectomy. Case report and review of literature. *Otolaryngol Pol.* 2014 Jul-Aug;68(4):204-7.

[58] Roh JL, Yoon YH, Park CI. Chyle leakage in patients undergoing thyroidectomy plus central neck dissection for differentiated papillary thyroid carcinoma. *Ann Surg Oncol.* 2008 Sep;15(9):2576-80.

[59] Rodier JF, Volkmar PP, Bodin F, Frigo S, Ciftci S, Dahlet C. Thoracic duct fistula after thyroid cancer surgery: towards a new treatment? *Case Rep Oncol.* 2011 May;4(2):255-9.

[60] Gosnell JE, Campbell P, Sidhu S, Sywak M, Reeve TS, Delbridge LW. Inadvertent tracheal perforation during thyroidectomy. . *Br J Surg* 2006;93:55–6.

[61] Damrose EJ, Damrose JF. Delayed tracheal rupture following thyroidectomy. *Auris Nasus Larynx.* 2009 Feb;36(1):113-5.

[62] Chauhan A, Ganguly M, Saidha N, Gulia P. Tracheal necrosis with surgical emphysema following thyroidectomy. *J Postgrad Med.* 2009 Jul-Sep;55(3):193-5.

[63] Bertolaccini L, Lauro C, Priotto R, Terzi A. It sometimes happens: late tracheal rupture after total thyroidectomy. *Interact Cardiovasc Thorac Surg.* 2012 Apr;14(4):500-1.

In: Thyroid Nodules
Editor: Marsha Vasquez
ISBN: 978-1-63483-592-3

Chapter VII

Diagnosis and Management of Thyroid Nodules Coexisting with Hashimoto's Thyroiditis: Pearls and Pitfalls

Mira Siderova**, *MD, PhD
University Hospital "St. Marina," Varna, Bulgaria
Department of Internal Medicine, Clinic of Endocrinology

Abstract

The association between Hashimoto's thyroiditis and differentiated thyroid cancer has been discussed in literature, but the relationship is still controversial. Coexistence of these two diseases is reported in up to 30% of cases, suggesting that there might be a pathological and causative link between them. On the other hand, the presence of thyroiditis may indicate a lower recurrence rate and a better prognosis of thyroid cancer. The diagnosis and follow-up in these cases may be challenging even for experts and require a wide range of laboratory, ultrasound (US), and morphology criteria in addition to an individualized approach.

In the background of Hashimoto's thyroiditis with the typical heterogeneous echotexture with hypoechoic micronodules and

* E-mail: mirasiderova@abv.bg.

hypervascularity, the sonographic appearance of a focal thyroid lesion may vary greatly, making it more difficult to differentiate between benign and malignant nodules, as well as between true nodules and pseudonodules. Fine needle aspiration biopsy is currently the best diagnostic test for the preoperative evaluation of thyroid nodules, including those coexistent with thyroiditis. However, the presence of lymphocytes and Hürthle cells may represent a potential source of error in cytological interpretation. Furthermore, there is an overlap in immunohistochemical staining and molecular profile between papillary carcinoma and Hashimoto's thyroiditis.

The aim of the present review is to summarize available evidence for the link between Hashimoto's thyroiditis and differentiated thyroid cancer with emphasis on US and cytology interpretation, the role of US elastography, and molecular markers. The promising use of thyroglobulin antibodies (TgAb) for postoperative monitoring of these patients will also be discussed.

Introduction

Hasimoto's thyroiditis (HT), also known as chronic lymphocytic or autoimmune thyroiditis, is the most common autoimmune thyroid disease and the most common cause of hypothyroidism [1]. It is associated with a characteristic sonographic appearance and circulating antibodies to thyroid antigens – thyroperoxidase (TPOAb) and thyroglobulin (TgAb). The disease was first described as a histologic diagnosis in 1912 by Hakaru Hashimoto, a Japanese surgeon and pathologist [2]. It occurs in 0,3-1,5 per 1000 individuals per year worldwide and is about 15 times more common in women than in men. Thyroid nodules are a very common clinical finding, with an estimated prevalence on the basis of palpation that ranges from 3% to 7% [3]. The widespread use of ultrasonography during the last decades has resulted in a dramatic increase in the prevalence of clinically inapparent thyroid nodules, estimated at 20% to 76% in the general population [4]. The prevalence of cancer reported for nonpalpable thyroid lesions ranges from 5.4% to 7.7% and appears to be similar to that reported for palpable lesions (5.0%- 6.5%) [5].

Hashimoto's thyroiditis and thyroid nodules commonly coexist in patients, thus fine needle aspiration biopsy (FNAB) is often employed to differentiate these two entities. The link between Hashimoto's thyroiditis and thyroid malignancy has long been a topic of controversy. There are conflicting reports; some suggest that these two are positively correlated, whereas other studies report no relationship.

Coexistence of Hashimoto's Thyroiditis with Differenciated Thyroid Carcinoma

The coexistence of Hashimoto's thyroiditis (HT) and differentiated thyroid carcinoma (DTC) was first described by Dailey et al. in 1955 [6]. Since then, numerous authors have reported coexistence of the two diseases, ranging from 0.5 to 30% [7-12, 15, 16, 19, 20, 22, 74]. Table 1 summarizes some of the biggest studies, belonging to one of the two main types of research: retrospective thyroidectomies and prospective cytology studies.

Table 1. Summary of retrospective and prospective studies on the coexistance of HT and DTC

First author/ year/reference	Study type	Study method	Number of patients	Females: Males	Prevalence of HT in DTC%
Kebebew, 2001 [10]	retrospective	Thyroidectomy	136	2.32:1	30
Cipolla, 2005 [9]	retrospective	Thyroidectomy	178	3:1	26.7
Repplinger, 2008 [8]	retrospective	Thyroidectomy	1198	3:1	29.0
Mazakopakis, 2010 [7]	retrospective	Thyroidectomy	140	6:1	28.57
Ahn, 2011 [74]	retrospective	Thyroidectomy	303	5.3:1	21.6
Jeong, 2012 [22]	retrospective	Thyroidectomy	1357	6.5:1	26.5
Holm, 1985 [16]	prospective	FNA	1658	15:1	0.12
Boi, 2005 [15]	prospective	FNA	590	9.4:1	13.7
Erdogan, 2009 [19]	prospective	FNA	769	16:1	0.52
Matesa-Anic, 2009 [20]	prospective	FNA	10508	9:1	1.95

The association between HT and DTC has been widely disputed and remains so in the literature, raising the following questions:

Which Type of Malignancy Is Associated with the Autoimmune Thyroiditis?

A well-established association that patients with chronic lymphocytic thyroiditis (CLT) have an increased risk of papillary thyroid carcinoma (PTC) and thyroid lymphoma has been proposed [13, 14]. Lee et al. analyzed sixteen studies investigating the frequencies of HT in PTCs and in other carcinomas such as follicular carcinoma and medullary carcinoma [13]. HT was present in 797 (17.1%) of 4664 PTC patients and in 57 (7.9%) of 725 other carcinoma patients [13]. The coexistence of HT was more related to PTCs than other thyroid carcinomas (OR 2.432; 95% CI 1.614–3.665; P<0.001).

In the study of Repplinger et al., papillary carcinomas were an overwhelming majority among the patients with Hashimoto's thyroiditis (94%) [8]. Although PTC was also the most common malignancy in patients without Hashimoto's thyroiditis (76%), it was significantly less common compared to patients with thyroiditis (p=0.001) [8].

Boi et al. compared the malignancy risk among antibody (ATA) positive and negative patients with nodular thyroid disease [15]. Regarding the type of thyroid cancer, the ATA negative group displayed PTC in 81.8% of patients and follicular thyroid carcinoma in 18.2% patients; in the ATA positive group almost all cases (96.3%) were PTC, assuming that there is a specific association between HT and PTC, rather than other thyroid tumor histotypes [15].

Thyroid lymphomas are rare diseases and almost always arise in the background of chronic lymphocytic thyroiditis. Among patients with Hashimoto's thyroiditis, the risk of thyroid lymphoma is at least 60 times higher than in patients without thyroiditis [16, 17]. Worldwide, the frequency of thyroid lymphoma appears to be higher in areas with a higher prevalence of thyroiditis. Most of thyroid lymphomas have B-cell origin and could be divided in two distinct clinical and prognostic subgroups [18]. The more indolent lymphomas are the subgroup of mucosa-associated lymphoid tissue (MALT) lymphomas comprising approximately 6% to 27% of thyroid lymphomas. This subgroup, when localized to the thyroid, responds well to total thyroidectomy or radiation with a complete response rate of more than 90%, leading some authors to recommend surgery as primary therapy in these cases [18]. Unfortunately, the more common subtype, comprising up to 70% of cases, is diffuse large B-cell lymphoma. This subtype appears to have the most aggressive clinical course with almost 60% of these tumors diagnosed with disseminated disease [18]. Treatment for these tumors should include chemotherapy and radiation. The overall 5-year survival for this aggressive group is less than 50%.

What Is the Prevalence of HT Among Patients with Thyroid Carcinoma?

This is illustrated in the so-called archival thyroidectomy studies, which analyze operated patients (mainly with already diagnosed by FNAB thyroid cancer) and calculate the frequency of HT among them. In a large meta-analysis performed by Lee [13] including 38 studies with 10 648 PTC cases, histologically proven HT was identified in 2471 (23.2%) of PTCs. HT was more frequently observed in PTCs than in benign thyroid diseases and other carcinomas (OR =2.8 and 2.4; P<0.001). PTCs with coexisting HT were significantly related to female patients (OR=2.7; P<0.001) and multifocal involvement (OR=1.5; P=0.010). Moreover, PTCs with HT were significantly associated with long recurrence-free survival (HR=0.6; P=0.001) [13].

The advantage of these archival thyroidectomy studies is that the diagnosis of both thyroid cancer and Hashimoto's thyroditis is based on strict histopathological criteria. Unfortunately they cannot explore the risk of PTC developing in patients with HT, because thyroiditis, as other benign thyroid diseases, is rarely an indication for surgery.

What Is the Prevalence of Thyroid Malignancy among Patients with Hashimoto's Thyroiditis?

In the last decade, much of the research exploring the relationship between HT and DTC has been done using fine-needle aspiration (FNA) cytology data that are more representative of a typical population of patients with HT [15, 19, 20]. Jankovic et al. conducted a recent literature review and found the prevalence of PTC in HT significantly lower among FNA specimens than in thyroidectomy specimens [21]. The average prevalence rate of PTC in patients with HT was 1.2% (ranged from 0.0 to 2.95) in eight FNA studies of 18,023 specimens and 27.6% (range, 9.5 to 36.6) in eight archival thyroidectomy studies of 9884 specimens [21]. The relative risk ratio of finding evidence of PTC in HT specimens ranged from 0.39 to 1.00 in the FNA group (average RR 0.69) in contrast to 1.15 to 4.16 from the archival thyroidectomy studies (average RR 1.59).

They concluded that the existing data provide inconsistent evidence favoring a causal relationship between HT and PTC [21]. Population-based studies using FNA cytology show no significant increase of PTC in patients with HT, whereas surgical series using thyroidectomy show a heightened risk for coexistent PTC, possibly related to selection bias. Prospective studies involving a large number of subjects and long-term follow-up are needed to further elucidate the relationship. Careful observation and follow-up of HT patients is recommended, especially those with nodular variants [21].

Clinical Manifestation and Prognostic Outcome

A number of investigators have reported that the presence of CLT in patients with PTC may be associated with different clinicopathological characteristics and may influence the prognostic outcome [13, 22, 23]. The main differences between the clinical presentation of PTC, with and without HT, concern age, gender, tumor size, multifocality, capsular invasion, extrathyroidal extension, and lymph node (LN) metastasis. Among the patients with coexistent PTC and CLT the prevalence of women is reported higher than in the group of PTC without CLT (96.7% vs. 83.1%, $p<0.0001$) [22]. At the time of the operation patients with PTC and CLT are younger than those only with PTC (44.5 vs 45.9 years, $p=0.047$). Mean tumor size is smaller in the cases with thyroiditis than in the cases without (17.9 vs 21.2 mm, $p=0.01$) [24]. According to some studies, up to 69% of the PTCs associated with HT are microcarcinomas (<1cm), and up to 77% are below 2 cm in diameter [25, 26]. Although of smaller size, thyroid malignancies with coexistent Hashimoto's thyroiditis have a tendency for multifocal involvement [10, 25, 27-29]. However, the coexistence of HT in PTCs is associated with a lower incidence of extrathyroidal invasion (OR=1.295; 95% CI 1.098–1.527; P=0.002) and a lower incidence of lymph node metastasis (OR=1.287; 95% CI 1.010–1.639; P=0.041), which can determine a less aggressive course and a better prognosis in these cases [13]. The presence of HT in PTCs is significantly associated with longer duration of recurrence-free survival and significantly lower recurrence rate during five-year follow-up (1.5% vs 5% in patients without HT, $p=0.042$) [22]. Patients with PTC and HT are less likely to receive additional treatment with radioiodine [24]. In contrast, other studies failed to present any beneficial effect of HT on the outcome of DTC [10, 26, 30].

What Is the Biological Explanation of the Link between HT and DTC?

Pathophysiological relationship between HT and DTC, in particular the papillary type, is still unclear, although three hypotheses have been proposed in the literature: (1) HT predisposes and facilitates the development of PTC, (2) HT is part of the host immune response against the tumor, or (3) HT is an incidental finding with concurrent PTC.

Chronic infection and inflammation contribute to around 25% of cancer cases worldwide [31]. While a direct link between several types of human malignancies and chronic inflammation has now been established, in particular for the gastrointestinal tract, the pathophysiology of chronic inflammation that induces papillary thyroid carcinoma (PTC) is still a subject of debate. At a molecular level, activation of the RET/PTC/RAS/BRAF/MAPK pathway, which induces both a pro-inflammatory and a pro-tumorigenic thyroid program, is a possible mechanism linking chronic inflammation with carcinogenesis [32, 33].

Sites of chronic inflammation are characterized by a rich lymphocyte, plasma cell, neutrophil, and macrophage infiltrate and by the production of a large amount of various cytokines, chemokines, growth factors, and oxygen and nitrogen reactive species [31, 34]. The latter may become deleterious in the context of an ongoing inflammatory process by generating highly mutagenic agents such as peroxynitrite, which cause point-mutations, rearrangements, and double-strand breaks in the DNA of proliferating epithelial and stroma cells [31]. This phenomenon is associated with an increased risk of oncogene activation and tumor suppressor gene loss of function which may lead to neoplastic transformation [31, 35]. Thus, the first hypothesis suggests a causative link, whereby the activated inflammatory response present in HT creates a favorable setting for malignant transformation of the thyroid epithelium.

In contrast, according to the second hypothesis, the lymphocytic infiltrate of HT may be an immunologic response with a cancer-retarding effect, contributing to a favorable outcome of PTC compared to other thyroid cancers. Presence of intratumoral or peritumoral infiltration of lymphocytes is evidence that the immune system may respond to malignant transformation. It is important to distinguish between diffuse (true CLT) and focal lymphocytic infiltration around the tumor [25]. However, Kebebew found a positive correlation between lymphocytic infiltration within or surrounding the tumor and the existence of CLT [10]. This may explain the "protective" effect of CLT in PTC.

Recent studies have reported that higher serum levels of TSH are associated with an increased incidence of thyroid malignancy in patients with nodular thyroid disease [36, 37]. However, different conditions including CLT may affect TSH concentration. A possible causative link between HT and DTC could be explained by elevated levels of TSH in subclinical and overt hypothyroid patients with HT, stimulating follicular epithelial proliferation, thereby promoting the development of papillary carcinoma [38].

Molecular Studies

In order to find a causative link between PTC and HT, many researchers have investigated the biomolecular profiles of the two conditions. At a molecular level, the RET/PTC/RAS/BRAF/MAPK pathway plays a critical role in thyroid cancer development and progression [39]. The MAPK cascade is a classical conserved intracellular signaling pathway involved in the regulation of cellular proliferation, differentiation, apoptosis and survival. Aberrant activation of the MAPK pathway, through activation of genetic alterations, has been found in numerous human malignancies, including thyroid cancer [31]. Physiologically, the tyrosine kinase membrane receptor RET can be stimulated by various growth factors and consecutively activates the membrane-bound G-protein RAS. RAS then interacts with and activates RAF protein kinase, which has three isoforms in mammals: A-RAF, B-RAF (BRAF) and C-RAF. In many cells, and particularly in thyroid follicular cells, BRAF is the most abundant and potent activator of the MAPK cascade [39]. Activated BRAF phosphorylates and activates MEK1 and MEK2, which in turn activate ERK 1 and ERK2. Finally, this process modifies the expression of various genes regulating key cellular functions such as proliferation, differentiation and apoptosis [39]. RET/PTC gene rearrangements are fusions between the 3' portion of the RET gene and the 5' portion of different unrelated genes, producing an aberrant RET/PTC protein with constitutive activation of the MAPK pathway. More than ten different fusion partners of

RET have been identified, the two most common types being *RET/PTC1* and *RET/PTC3*. They are found in 20–40% of adult sporadic papillary carcinomas and with higher prevalence in children and in patients exposed to radiation [40].

Several authors have found *RET/PTC* rearrangements in nonneoplastic thyroid lesions, such as CLT [41-43]. Muzza et al. investigated clinical and molecular features of 128 patients with PTC and concurrent CLT and 215 patients with PTC alone [42]. The two groups did not show significant differences in clinical and prognostic findings, whereas they harboured a significantly different genetic background, with *RET/PTC1* being more represented in PTCs associated with autoimmunity and *BRAF (V600E)* in patients with PTC alone. Interestingly, *RET/PTC1* rearrangement was also found in 41% of nonneoplastic thyroid cells, contralateral to the tumors. The strong association between *RET/PTC1* and thyroiditis points to a critical role of this oncoprotein in the modulation of the autoimmune response [42].

Rhoden et al. investigated samples of both CLT and PTC, using two detection techniques, interphase fluorescence *in situ* hybridization (FISH) and RT-PCR [43]. They found that low-level *RET/PTC* recombination occurs in nonneoplastic follicular cells in CLT and in a subset of PTC, suggesting that overlapping molecular mechanisms may govern early stages of tumor development and inflammation in the thyroid [43]. However, according to other authors using this ultrasensitive RT-PCR technique could result in abundance of false-positive cases and should be interpreted with caution [40].

The most common of *BRAF* mutations is a point mutation at residue 600 of the BRAF protein called the *BRAFV600E* mutation and occurs in approximately 45% of patients with PTC. Although its role as a prognostic factor is still controversial, recent studies have shown that patients with a BRAF mutation may be more likely to have clinicopathologic characteristics of more aggressive disease, such as extrathyroidal invasion, lymph node metastasis, and advanced tumor stage at initial surgery. Kim et al. found that in Korean patients with papillary carcinoma *BRAF(V600E)* mutation is associated with a lower frequency of background HT [44]. As mentioned above, BRAF activating mutations are rarely encountered in HT-associated PTCs, where the RET/PTC rearrangement is the most frequent genetic alteration. This could explain the better prognosis of the coexistence of the two entities.

Larson et al. [45] found that PI3K pathway components that are known to be involved in carcinogenesis (specifically phosphorylated-Akt, Akt1, and Akt2) are expressed in PTC and in HT (within infiltrating lymphocytes), whereas they are not expressed in normal surrounding thyroid tissue. Interestingly, higher levels of PI3K/Akt expression were found when HT was associated with PTC, than in PTC alone. In contrast, tumor suppressor gene, PTEN, was expressed in normal thyroid specimens. PTEN was also expressed in HT specimens, especially within infiltrating lymphocytes and areas of Hürthle cell changes, whereas there was minimal expression of PTEN in papillary carcinoma cells [45].

Anderson et al. [46] demonstrated that the expression of CD98, a component of a cell surface amino acid transporter, was decreased in inflamed areas of both HT and PTC compared to normal follicular cells, follicular adenoma or carcinoma, multinodular goiter and Grave's disease. Since CD98 activates β1-integrin, thus promoting anchorage-independent growth, they concluded that this down-regulation of CD98 could explain, in part, the good prognosis of PTC, particularly in the context of HT [46].

Diagnostic Dilemmas and the Role of US in the Preoperative Detection of Thyroid Carcinoma in the Setting of Hashimoto's Thyroiditis

Over the last few decades, ultrasonography has become an indispensable tool for the diagnosis of thyroid diseases, in particular thyroid nodules and has had a profound impact on the improved patient care [47]. The diagnosis of autoimmune thyroiditis is usually based on laboratory tests and, less frequently, on symptoms or signs [48, 49]. Prior studies have reported that autoantibodies are absent in 13% and are low in 17% of patients with Hashimoto's thyroiditis and are present in 2–20% of the population without thyroid disease [50]. In fact, if only clinical and serum findings were used to diagnose HT, the diagnosis would be missed in at least half of patients [51]. The sensitivity and specificity improve dramatically by combining ultrasound evaluation with clinical and serological assessments [50, 51]. The diagnostic role of US is especially important in detecting thyroid nodules in the setting of autoimmune thyroiditis.

The sonographic appearance of Hashimoto's thyroiditis is well recognized and is described as hypoechoic, heterogeneous and hypervascular parenchyma with micronodulation and echogenic septations [52]. Usually, the gland is diffusely enlarged, but often the size is normal or even decreased in the atrophic variant. The micronodules range from about 1 to 7 mm in size and correspond to focal lymphocytic infiltration, whereas the echogenic septations occur secondary to fibrosis inside the parenchyma (Figure 1A). This micronodular pattern on ultrasound is highly diagnostic of Hashimoto's thyroiditis with a positive predictive value of 95% [53]. The increased vascularity on color doppler seems to be associated with the development of hypothyroidism, which may be due to the trophic stimulation of thyroid-stimulating hormone [54].

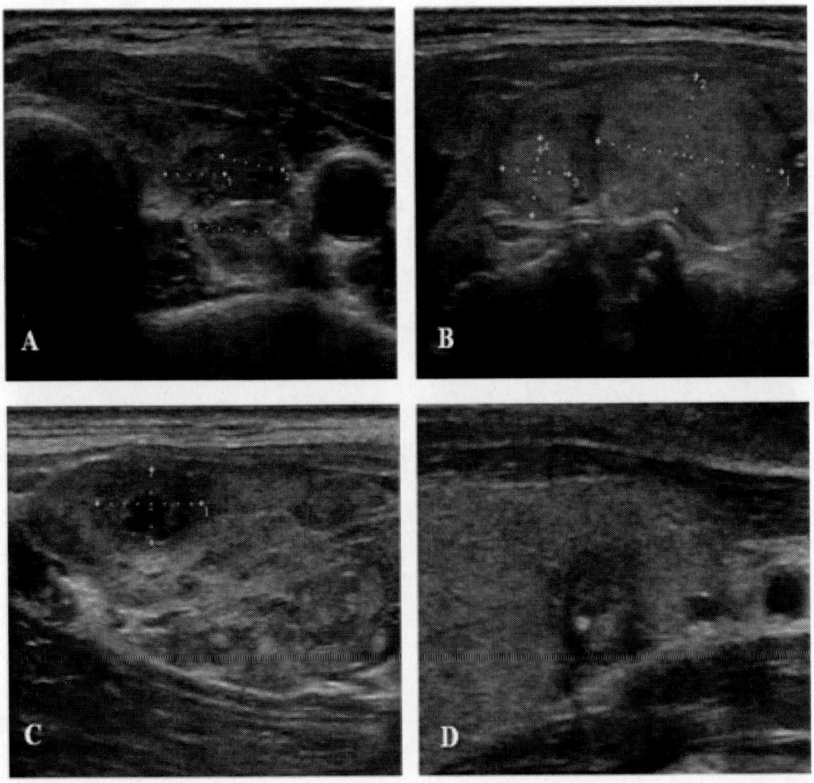

Figure 1. A. US image of Hashimoto's thyroiditis with echogenic septations and formation of pseudonodules, cytologically proven to be lymphocytic infiltrates; B. Nodular form of Hashimoto's thyroiditis presented as hyperechoic nodules; C. A mixed nodule with ill defined ventral margins on the background of Hashimoto's thyroiditis, benign on cytology; D. Hypoechoic taller-than-wide nodule with ill defined margins and grouped microcalcifications, papillary carcinoma on cytology and histology.

The nodular form of Hashimoto's thyroiditis, also known as focal thyroiditis, or pseudotumor, is usually confirmed on cytology after FNAB [55]. According to previous studies the nodular form comprises approximately 5% of all biopsied nodules [52, 55]. Some authors have suggested that nodular thyroiditis is an early presentation of Hashimoto's thyroiditis [56]. Others think, however, that it is a completely different clinical form of Hashimoto's thyroiditis [9]. In addition, true nodules may also occur within diffusely altered parenchyma or within sonographically normal parenchyma. The extremely variable US image in such cases (Figure 1A,B,C,D) raises the following questions:

- Is this a nodule or a pseudonodule?
- Is the nodule benign or malignant?
- What kind of noninvasive or invasive diagnostic methods should we apply to answer these questions?

No strict criteria have been established to differentiate nodules from pseudonodules. A nodule is defined as an intrathyroidal lesion of any size that is sonographically distinct from the surrounding thyroid tissue – purely demarcated or vascularized differently (less or more than native parenchyma). If a lesion is not demarcated in B-mode or color doppler it is usually referred as a pseudonodule [57].

In a multiinstitutional study, Anderson et al. analyzed the sonographic appearance of 64 cases of nodular Hashimoto's thyroiditis, confirmed to be lymphocytic thyroiditis on cytology [52]. The mean diameter of nodular Hashimoto's thyroiditis was 15 ± 7.33 mm. It occurred as a solitary nodule in 36% of cases and in the setting of five or more nodules in 23% of cases. Fifty-five percent of the cases of nodular Hashimoto thyroiditis occurred within a sonographic background of diffuse Hashimoto's thyroiditis, and 45% of cases occurred within normal thyroid parenchyma [52]. The sonographic appearance was extremely variable. Within a background of diffuse Hashimoto's thyroiditis, nodular Hashimoto's thyroiditis was more likely to be a solid lesion, to be hyperechoic, to have a thin regular hypoechoic halo, to have no calcifications, and to occur as a solitary nodule. On the other hand, nodular Hashimoto's thyroiditis within normal thyroid parenchyma was more likely to have some cystic elements and to have peripheral eggshell calcifications. Nodular Hashimoto's thyroiditis within normal parenchyma was also more likely to have additional focal nodules. Of these differences, only solid composition was statistically significant [52]. According to the authors, some of these trends could be explained. In patients with diffuse CLT, all nodules should be expected to display a higher echogenicity when compared with the hypoechoic background parenchyma. This idea may at least partially explain why nodular Hashimoto thyroiditis was more hyperechoic in the setting of diffuse Hashimoto's thyroiditis than when it was within an otherwise normal gland [52, 55]. The heterogeneous nature of diffuse CLT can also make nodules harder to identify and may explain why nodular Hashimoto's thyroiditis was more often solitary in the setting of diffuse thyroiditis than in the setting of a normal-appearing background parenchyma (51% vs 17%). Nevertheless, due to fact that the US features were extremely variable and overlapped with the findings typically associated with other benign nodules as well as malignant nodules, this study failed to determine a "typical" sonographic appearance for nodular Hashimoto's thyroiditis [52].

As a part of the same multiinstitutional study, Anderson et al. compared sonographic features of benign and malignant nodules in patients with diffuse Hashimoto's thyroiditis [58]. The mean diameter of malignant nodules (12,7 mm) was smaller than benign (15,6 mm), although the difference was not statistically significant. Malignant nodules were more likely to be solid and hypoechoic (62% vs 19%). All types of calcifications were more prevalent among malignant nodules, including microcalcifications (39% vs 0%), macrocalcifications (15% vs 3%), and eggshell calcifications (15% vs 2%). Benign nodules were more likely to be hyperechoic (46% vs 9%), to have a halo (39% vs 15%), and to lack calcifications (88% vs 23%). Color doppler examination showed variable vascularity with a similar proportion of benign and malignant nodules being hypervascular, isovascular, hypovascular, and avascular. The variability in vascularity may be partially explained by the fact that the thyroid parenchyma in patients with diffuse Hashimoto's thyroiditis is often hypervascular, which would tend to alter the impression of vascularity in focal nodules [58].

Thus, the US features of benign and malignant nodules within diffuse Hashimoto's thyroiditis are generally similar to the features typical of benign and malignant nodules in the general population. If calcifications of any type are added to the list of malignant sonographic features, the decision to biopsy a nodule in patients with diffuse Hashimoto's thyroiditis can be based on recommendations that have been published previously [58]. Unfortunately, some signs that may help in the general population, such as margin characteristics and vascularity, do not seem to be as useful in patients with diffuse Hashimoto's thyroiditis. Therefore, the percentage of benign nodules that require biopsy is likely to be higher in patients with HT than in patients with sonographically normal thyroid parenchyma [58].

US Elastography

Fine needle aspiration biopsy (FNAB) is the gold standard in the preoperative management of focal lesions on the background of Hashimoto's thyroiditis, classifing them as either true nodules (benign, malignant, indeterminate or suspicious on cytology) or pseudonodules (inflammatory changes due to the thyroiditis). Despite its accuracy for diagnosis, FNAB is categorized as a minimally invasive intervention.

In contrast, sonoelastography is a noninvasive dynamic technique that uses US to provide an estimation of tissue stiffness by measuring the degree of distortion under the application of an external force. US elastography has been applied to study the hardness/elasticity of nodules to differentiate malignant from benign lesions [59, 60]. Real Time Ultrasound Elastography (RTE) is in most commonly used in thyroid clinics. The nodule chosen by the operator and taken in to the area of interest, is subjected to repeated pressure pulses applied by the probe; pressure is standardized and displayed as pressure scores from 1 to 6, or in between the diagrams on the screen. Optimally, the pressure pulses are kept between 3 to 4 during the examination. Tissue distortion is then processed by a special software and presented an US elastogram over the B-mode image in a color scale that ranges from red, for components with greatest elastic strain (i.e., softest components), to blue for those with no strain (i.e., hardest components). The US elastographic image is then matched with an elasticity color scale and classified using an elasticity scoring system [59, 61, 62]. Figure 2 presents elasticity scoring for thyroid nodules modified from Ito by Rago [59], as well as conventional US and RTE of five different thyroid nodules. Rago further simplified the score in three categories – high, intermediate and low elasticity [63].

A strain index (SI) could be calculated as a ratio of the nodule strain divided by the strain of the softest part of the surrounding normal tissue. The cut-off of SI for malignancy was estimated to be 2.9 in a study of Magri in 661 nodules [64]. Others proposed a higher cut-off of 3.85 for detecting malignant thyroid nodules [65].

Having in mind that the surrounding parenchyma in HT is usually with lower elasticity, especially in areas of fibrosis [66], there are some concerns about the diagnostic accuracy of RTE in distinguishing true nodules from pseudonodules, as well as benign from malignant lesions in the settings of Hashimoto's thyroiditis.

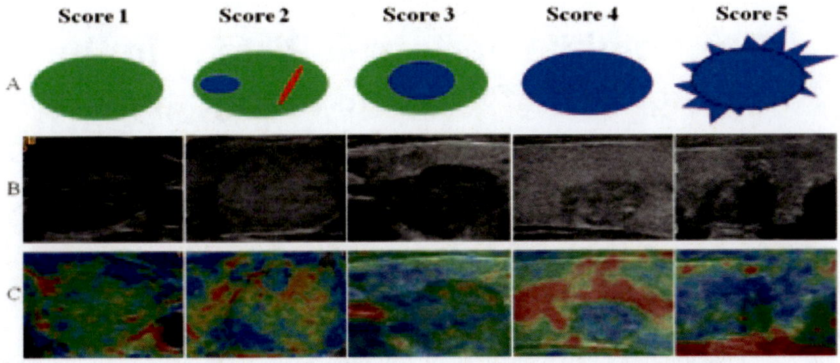

Figure 2 A. Elasticity scoring scale: score 1 - elasticity in the whole nodule; score 2 – elasticity in a large part of the nodule; score 3 – elasticity only at the periphery of the nodule; score 4 – no elasticity in the nodule; score 5 – no elasticity in the nodule and part of the surrounding tissue; B. Conventional US in B-mode of five different thyroid nodules C. Elastography of the same five nodules.

Based on the results from RTE in 54 focal lesions with coexistent HT, Yildirim proposes if the lesion is isoelastic with the surrounding tissue, it should be referred as a pseudonodule. If the elasticity of the focal lesion is different (greater or lesser than the basal parenchymal elasticity and occupies ≥ 50% of the surface area of the nodule itself), it should be categorized as a true nodule [57]. Comparison between conventional B-mode US and FNAB gave a correlation of 54.4% between the two methods in distinguishing nodules from pseudonodules, whereas sonoelastography versus FNAB demonstrated a correlation of 85.9%. Moreover, elastography increased the sensitivity of US examination from 85.7% to 92.9%, specificity from 77.5% to 95.0%, and accuracy from 79.6% to 94.4%, respectively. Thus, this new noninvasive technique is able to detect true nodules often misdiagnosed by conventional grey scale US [57]. On the other hand, the increase in specificity may avoid useless biopsies of pseudonodules.

The diagnostic value of real time elastography in distinguishing benign from malignant nodules on the background of HT was assessed in 283 patients by Sahin et al. [67]. According to their results, an elastography score ≥ 3 provides 80% sensitivity and 50% specificity for diagnosing malignancy, whereas a strain index with a cut-off of ≥ 2.45 shows 72.2% sensitivity and

70% specificity. Since Hashimoto's thyroiditis changes the hardness of the surrounding tissue, strain index reflects malignancy better than the elasticity score.

Morphology Pearls and Pitfalls in the Diagnose of Thyroid Malignancy Accompanied by Hashimoto's Thyroiditis

Nodules and pseudonodules are frequent in Hashimoto's thyroiditis and are a common indication for *FNAB*. Aspirates of chronic lymphocytic thyroiditis are characterized by a combination of two features: (1) a mixed population of lymphocytes, plasma cells, and lymphohistiocytic aggregates, and (2) occasional cohesive clusters of follicular cells with oncocytic features, called Hürthle cells [68]. Potential pitfalls can result from cytologic atypia occurring in autoimmune thyroiditis; abundance or scarcity of background inflammation; low cell yield; and co-existing toxicity and malignancies [69]. The smaller size of papillary carcinomas, usually microcarcinomas, and the fibrotic changes in the surrounding parenchyma with CLT may cause technical difficulties in performing the FNAB. Thus, a neoplasm can be overlooked based on inadequate cell sampling in a biopsy from HT, resulting in false-negative diagnosis [69]. On the contrary, follicular cell changes, especially the oncocytic changes associated with HT can be mistaken for a neoplasm leading to false-positive diagnosis [70]. Oncocytes, also called "Hürthle" cells are characterised by abundant eosinophilic granular cytoplasm as a result of the accumulation of altered mitochondria. This is a phenomenon of metaplasia that occurs in inflammatory disorders, such as thyroiditis, or other situations that result in cellular stress [71]. On the other hand, the same Hürthle cells, although like a predominant cell type in the aspirate, are seen in Hürthle cell adenomas and carcinomas, as well as in oxyphilic variant of PTC. Another pitfall in cytology is due to the fact that follicular cells associated with the lymphocytic infiltrate may show clearing of the nuclear chromatin and grooves, which may be mistaken for papillary carcinoma [72]. Occasionally the dense lymphoid component in CLT can be difficult to differentiate from a low-grade lymphoplasmacytoid lymphoma [73]. Most of the mentioned examples of difficult cases in thyroid pathology may require the use of ancillary techniques as immunohistochemistry and molecular diagnostics.

On histology, HT is characterized by diffuse lymphocytic and plasma cell infiltrate, Hürthle cells, and the formation of lymphoid follicles and reactive germinal centers. In cases of coexistence of DTC and HT the infiltrate must be present also in the thyroid tissue, distinct from the site of the carcinoma [74]. Non-specific lymphocytic infiltration occurring immediately adjacent to the tumor may represent perineoplastic inflammation and should not be considered true HT to avoid overdiagnosis [25]. The most common thyroid cancer – PTC is diagnosed based on the presence of distinctive nuclear features, including overlapping and elongation of the nuclei, clear "ground glass" nuclei with hypodense chromatin, nuclear grooves and pseudoinclusions, as well as the formation of neoplastic papillae and the presence of psammoma bodies. Follicular carcinoma (FC) is diagnosed when either capsular or vascular invasion or both are present.

As mentioned above, small tumoral size (usually microcarcinomas) and multifocality are common characteristics of PTC in the background of HT. Di Pasquale et al. analyzed the morphology of Hashimoto's associated thyroid carcinomas in order to find out whether these tumors show any other distinctive histological features [75]. 67% of the PTC with coexistent HT showed various degree of intratumoral fibrosis, ranging from thick fibrous septa separating tumor nodules to almost complete obliteration of the tumor by the fibrosis, with only microscopic residual tumor nests. All the tumors, independently of the degree of fibrosis, showed the nuclear features of PTC. No correlation was found between the degree of fibrosis in the tumors and the thyroid gland outside the tumors, there were even tumors with marked internal fibrosis without fibrosis outside the tumor [75]. Another finding of their study was the presence of a pseudovascular pattern of tumor growth, characrerized by cystic spaces with hyalinized walls and focal papillary hyperplasia lined by flat and cuboidal epithelium. Thus, the diagnosis of PTC may be missed if the cells lining the spaces are not examined at higher magnification and the nuclear features of PTC are not identified [75]. An important differential diagnosis with this angiomatoid pattern is the reactive vascular hyperplasia that has been described in adenomatous goiter of the thyroid [76].

Although conventional histology is the diagnostic cornerstone of thyroid malignancy, *immunohistochemical techniques* detecting expression of some molecular markers can be an useful adjunct. A variety of molecular markers are abnormally expressed in malignant thyroid tumors and are not commonly found in benign lesions. These molecules are involved in different biological processes (cell transformation, proliferation, differentiation, metastasis, resistance to apoptosis) and are associated with tumor initiation and progression [77]. Galectin-3 is beta-galactoside binding polypeptide, expressed mainly in the cytoplasm and nuclei of malignant follicular cells [78]. Galectin-3 regulates the cell cycle by inhibiting apoptosis and stimulating cell proliferation.

As an adhesion molecule detected on the cell surface and in the extracellular matrix, it participates in different stages of tumor progression and metastasis. Fibronectin-1 is an extracellular matrix protein, produced by fibroblasts. Its cytoplasmic positivity in thyroid follicular cells is associated with their malignant transformation [79]. Cytokeratin-19 is a low molecular weight cytokeratin with strong and diffuse cytoplasmic expression in malignant thyroid cells [80]. The cell surface mesothelial antigen, which is recognized by the monoclonal antibody HBME1, indicates malignancy but not papillary differentiation [81]. An antibody panel consisting of galectin-3, cytokeratin-19, HBME1, and fibronectin-1 might contribute to differential diagnosis between malignant and benign thyroid lesions, since their expression is strong and diffuse in PTC, follicular variant of PTC (FVPTC), FC, Hürthle cell carcinoma, and anaplastic carcinoma, whereas normal thyroid tissue and benign lesions do not show immunopositivity [77]. Immunohistochemistry offers diagnostic advantages in cases of cystic thyroid lesions that can harbor occult papillary carcinoma [82], in less differentiated variants and in lymph node metastases [77]. Intrathyroidal microfoci of PTC are better visualized by IHH and distinguished from benign hyperplastic changes with papillization [83].

The diagnosis of microcarcinomas, especially below 5 mm, and multifocality of the tumor is often clear after immunohistochemical analysis [77]. Since microcarcinomas and multifocality are common features of Hashimoto's associated thyroid malignancy, IHH appears to be a useful diagnostic tool. On the other hand, there are reports that focal PTC-like immunopositivity for galectin 3, CITED1, cytokeratin 19 (CK19), HBME1 and fibronectin-1 expression may be found in HT, suggesting the possibility of early, focal premalignant transformation of follicular epitelium in some cases of HT [79].

The expression of these markers, mainly CK19, is weak and focal, limited to areas of cystic degeneration, chronic inflammation and lymphocytic infiltration [84] in contrast to diffuse positivity in PTC, FVPTC and anaplastic cancer which has diagnostic value [85].

Follow up of Patients with DTC and Coexistent HT

Not only diagnosis, but also follow up of patients with differentiated thyroid carcinoma is more difficult with coexistent autoimmunity. The past 20 years have witnessed a major paradigm shift in the methods used to detect postoperative recurrence, with a clear decline in the use of whole body scans and increasingly widespread reliance on high-resolution ultrasound with serum thyroglobulin (Tg) examination after initial surgical intervention [86]. Ultrasound has proved to be more accurate than whole body scanning for detecting recurrent/persistent disease in low-risk DTC patients [87, 88]. Serum Tg is considered the most sensitive marker for the presence of DTC after total thyroidectomy and radioactive iodine (RAI) treatment, especially when thyrotropin (TSH) is elevated through thyroid hormone withdrawal or injection of recombinant human TSH (rhTSH). The presence of circulating thyroglobulin antibodies (TgAb) in patients with DTC and HT, however, may limit the use of serum thyroglobulin as a primary tumor marker due to methodological problems in the determination of serum thyroglobulin. Tg-immunoradiometric assay (IRMA) are more influenced and can underestimate serum Tg concentration, while Tg-radioimmunoassay (RIA) are less prone to TgAb interference, but may overestimate Tg levels [89]. Underestimation of serum Tg in TgAb positive sera is the most serious type of interference with clinical significance, as this may mask the presence of recurrent or persistent thyroid carcinoma. However, in such cases serial TgAb measurements may be used as a surrogate marker for recurrence of thyroid cancer during the long-term monitoring of DTC patients [90].

Based on recent studies it was proposed that serial TgAb measurements could have a prognostic significance for monitoring response to DTC treatment [90, 91]. Patients who have persistent disease after initial treatment retain detectable TgAb concentrations [90, 91]. A rise in TgAb level is often the first indication of recurrence in such patients [92]. In a review on autoimmunity in DTC, Rasmussen et al. also recommend measurement of serum TgAb as an adjunct to Tg in the follow-up of DTC. Thus, persistently elevated TgAb levels appear to serve as a useful marker for recurrent or persistent DTC in patients with undetectable serum thyroglobulin levels while decreasing titers is favourable [90]. In a study of Chung et al. 22.6% of Tg undetectable patients showed positive TgAb, and in 49% of them recurrence was confirmed [89]. TgAb-positive patients showed a higher recurrence rate than that of TgAb-negative patients ($p<0.0001$). Moreover, during follow up 73.1% of the disease-free patients showed spontaneously decreased TgAb levels [89]. In a study of Chiovato et al. the median disappearance time of TgAb after initial treatment (thyroidectomy and Iodine-131) was 3.0 years [93]. Clearly, it is the trend in TgAb concentrations that is more significant than any single TgAb concentration per se. This was apparent from the 2008 study by Kim et. al.which found that less than 1% of patients who became TgAb-negative or displayed more than a 50% decline in TgAb over the 6 to 12 months after radioiodine treatment had a recurrence detected during follow-up [94]. In contrast, 19% of patients in whom TgAb declined less than 50%, as well as the 37% in whom TgAb concentrations rose, were diagnosed with recurrences [94]. It should be noted that a rising TgAb trend or a de novo appearance of TgAb is commonly seen in the first few months following radioiodine therapy or fine-needle aspiration biopsy in response to Tg antigen released by damaged cells. These responses tend to be transient (1–8 months) and should be distinguished from a sustained, progressive TgAb rise, or sustained de novo appearance of TgAb, that may be an early indicator of recurrence [95].

In conclusion, the diagnosis of thyroid cancer in the presence of thyroiditis is very difficult. It is important to make a careful examination and follow-up of patients with HT and in cases of suspected nodules to use all advances in technology as US elastography and FNAB with ancillary techniques. Despite the better prognosis for PTC with coexistent HT, the initial treatment comprised of surgery and radioiodine according to risk stratification does not differ from general recommendations for DTC. The clinician should also be aware of the pitfalls of Tg measurement in the postoperative follow up of patients with DTC and thyroid autoimmunity. Although TgAbs interfere with Tg measurements, TgAb concentration trends can be used as a surrogate DTC tumor marker.

References

[1] Pearce EN, Farwell AP, Braveman LE. Thyroiditis. *N Engl J Med* 2003; 348(26):2646-2655.

[2] Hashimoto H. Zur Kenntniss der lymphomatösen Veränderung der Schilddrüse (Struma lymphomatosa). *Arch Klin Chir* 1912; 97: 219-248.

[3] Hegedüs L. Clinical practice. The thyroid nodule. *N Engl J Med* 2004; 351(17):1764-1771 .

[4] Ezzat S, Sarti DA, Cain DR, Braunstein GD. Thyroid incidentalomas: Prevalence by palpation and ultrasonography. *Arch Intern Med* 1994; 154(16):1838-1840.

[5] Gharib H, Papini E, Paschke R, Duick DS, Valcavi R, Hegedüs L, Vitti P. AACE/AME/ETA Medical guidelines for clinical practice for the diagnosis and management of thyroid nodules. *Endocr Pract* 2010; 16 (Suppl 1): 1-42.

[6] Dailey ME, Lindsay S, Skahen R. Relation of thyroid neoplasms to Hashimoto disease of the thyroid gland. *AMA Arch Surg* 1955; 70(2):291–297.

[7] Mazokopakis EE, Tzortzinis AA, Dalieraki-Ott EI, Tsartsalis AN, Syros PK, Karefilakis CM, Papadomanolaki MG, Starakis IK. Coexistence of Hashimoto's thyroiditis with papillary thyroid carcinoma. A retrospective study. *Hormones* 2010; 9(4):312-317.

[8] Repplinger D, Bargren A, Zhang YW, Adler J, Haymart M, Chen H. Is Hashimoto's thyroiditis a risk factor for papillary thyroid cancer? *J Surg Res* 2008; 150(1):49–52.

[9] Cipolla C, Sandonato L, Graceffa G, , Fricano S, Torcivia A, Vieni S, Latteri S, Latteri MA. Hashimoto's thyroiditis coexistent with papillary thyroid carcinoma. *Am Surg* 2005; 71(10): 874-878.

[10] Kebebew E, Treseler PA, Ituarte PH, Clark OH. Coexisting chronic lymphocytic thyroiditis and papillary thyroid cancer revisited. *World J Surg* 2001; 25(5):632-7.

[11] Konturek A, Barczyński M, Wierzchowski W, Stopa M, Nowak W. Coexistence of papillary thyroid cancer with Hashimoto thyroiditis. *Langenbecks Arch Surg* 2013; 398(3):389–394.

[12] Singh B, Shaha AR, Trivedi H, Carew JF, Poluri A, Shah JP. Coexistent Hashimoto's thyroiditis with papillary thyroid carcinoma: impact on presentation, management, and outcome. *Surgery* 1999; 126(6):1070-6; discussion 1076-7.

[13] Lee JH, Kim Y, Choi JW, Kim YS. The association between papillary thyroid carcinoma and histologically proven Hashimoto's thyroiditis: a meta-analysis. *Eur J Endocrinol* 2013; 168(3): 343–349 .

[14] Moshynska OV, Saxena A. Clonal relationship between Hashimoto thyroiditis and thyroid lymphoma. *J Clin Pathol* 2008; 61(4):438-444 .

[15] Boi F, Lai ML, Marziani B, Minerba L, Faa G and Mariotti S. High prevalence of suspicious cytology in thyroid nodules associated with

positive thyroid autoantibodies. *European Journal of Endocrinology* 2005; 153 (5) 637–642.

[16] Holm L-E, Blomgren H, Lowhagen T. Cancer risks in patients with chronic lymphocytic thyroiditis. *N Engl J Med* 1985;312(10):601–4.

[17] Pedersen RK, Pedersen NT. Primary non-Hodgkin's lymphoma of the thyroid gland: a population based study. *Histopathology* 1996; 28(1):25-32.

[18] Widder S, Pasieka JL. Primary thyroid lymphoma. *Curr Treat Options Oncol* 2004; 5(4): 307-13.

[19] Erdogan M, Erdem N, Cetinkalp S, et al. Demographic, clinical, laboratory, ultrasonographic, and cytological features of patients with Hashimoto's thyroiditis: a result of a university hospital of 769 patients in Turkey. *Endocrine* 2009; 36(3):486–490..

[20] Matesa-Anic′ D, Matesa N, Dabelic′ N, Kusic′ Z. Coexistence of papillary carcinoma and Hashimoto's thyroiditis. *Acta Clin Croat* 2009; 48(1):9–12..

[21] Jankovic B, Le KT, Hershman JM. Clinical Review: Hashimoto's thyroiditis and papillary thyroid carcinoma: is there a correlation? *J Clin Endocrinol Metab* 2013; 98(2):474-82.

[22] Jeong JS, Kim HK, Lee CR, Park S, Park JH, Kang SW, Jeong JJ, Nam KH, Chung WY, Park CS. Coexistence of Chronic Lymphocytic Thyroiditis with Papillary Thyroid Carcinoma: Clinical Manifestation and Prognostic Outcome. *J Korean Med Sci* 2012; 27(8):883-889.

[23] Hershman JM. Patients with Differentiated Thyroid Cancer and Coexistent Hashimoto's Thyroiditis Have a Better Prognosis Than Those without Thyroiditis. *Clin Thyroidol* 2013; 25(10):225–226.

[24] Dvorkin S, Robenshtok E, Hirsch D, Strenov Y, Shimon I, Benbassat CA. Differentiated thyroid cancer is associated with less aggressive disease and better outcome in patients with coexisting Hashimotos thyroiditis. *J Clin Endocrinol Metab* 2013; 98(6):2409-14.

[25] Hristozov KH, Siderova MV, Krasnaliev IJ, Nenkov R, Radev R. Is there a difference in tumor size and number of foci in Hashimoto's associated thyroid cancer? *Eur Thyroid J* 2012; 1(suppl 1): 145 .

[26] Zhang Y, Ma XP, Deng FS et al. The effect of chronic lymphocytic thyroiditis on patients with thyroid cancer. *World J Surg Oncol* 2014; 12(1): 277; doi:10.1186/1477-7819-12-277.

[27] Kim KW, Park YJ, Kim EH, Park SY, Park do J, Ahn SH, Jang HC, Cho BY. Elevated risk of papillary thyroid cancer in Korean patients with Hashimoto's thyroiditis. *Head & Neck* 2011; 33(5): 691–695.

[28] Consorti F, Loponte M, Milazzo F, Potasso L, Antonaci A. Risk of malignancy from thyroid nodular disease as an element of clinical management of patients with Hashimoto's thyroiditis. *European Surgical Research* 2010; 45(3-4):333–337.

[29] Gul K, Dirikoc A, Kiyak G, Ersoy PE, Ugras NS, Ersoy R, Cakir B. The association between thyroid carcinoma and Hashimoto's thyroiditis: the ultrasonographic and histopathologic characteristics of malignant nodules. *Thyroid* 2010, 20(8): 873-878; doi:10.1089/thy.2009.0118..

[30] Kim HG, Kim EK, Han KH et al. Pathologic Spectrum of Lymphocytic Infiltration and Recurrence of Papillary Thyroid Carcinoma. *Yonsei Med J* 2014; 55(4):879-885.

[31] Bozec A, Lassalle S, Hofman V, Ilie M, Santini J, Hofman P. The Thyroid Gland: A Crossroad in Inflammation-Induced Carcinoma? An Ongoing Debate with New Therapeutic Potential. *Current Medicinal Chemistry* 2010; 17(30):3449-3461.

[32] Russell, J.P.; Engiles, J.B.; Rothstein, J.L. Proinflammatory mediators and genetic background in oncogene mediated tumor progression. *J Immunol* 2004; 172(7):4059-4067, doi: 10.4049/jimmunol.172.7.4059.

[33] Russell, J.P.; Shinohara, S.; Melillo, R.M.; Castellone, M.D.; Santoro, M.; Rothstein, J.L. Tyrosine kinase oncoprotein, RET/PTC3, induces the secretion of myeloid growth and chemotactic factors. *Oncogene* 2003; 22(29): 4569-4577.

[34] Hussain, S.P.; Harris, C.C. Inflammation and cancer: an ancient link with novel potentials. *Int J Cancer* 2007; 121(11):2373-2380.

[35] Lu H, Ouyang W, Huang C. Inflammation, a key event in cancer development. *Mol Cancer Res* 2006; 4(4): 221-233.

[36] Boelaert K, Horacek J, Holder RL, Watkinson JC, Sheppard MC, Franklyn JA. Serum thyrotropin concentration as a novel predictor of malignancy in thyroid nodules investigated by fine needle aspiration. *J Clin Endocrinol Metab* 2006; 91(11):4295– 4301.

[37] Fiore E, Vitti P. Serum TSH and risk of papillary thyroid cancer in nodular thyroid disease. *J Clin Endocrinol Metab* 2012; 97(4):1134-45.

[38] McLeod DS, Watters KF, Carpenter AD, Ladenson PW, Cooper DS, Ding EL. Thyrotropin and thyroid cancer diagnosis: a systematic review and dose-response meta-analysis. *J Clin Endocrinol Metab* 2012; 97(8):2682–2692..

[39] Xing M. BRAF mutation in papillary thyroid cancer: pathogenic role, molecular bases, and clinical implications. *Endocr Rev* 2007; 28(7):742-762.

[40] Nikiforov Y. RET/PTC rearrangement – a link between Hashimoto's thyroiditis and thyroid cancer...or not. *J Clin Endocrinol Metab* 2006; 91(6):2040-2042.

[41] Wirtschafter A , Schmidt R , Rosen D, Kundu N, Santoro M, Fusco A, Multhaupt H, Atkins JP, Rosen MR, Keane WM, Rothstein JL. Expression of the R ET/PTC fusion gene as a marker of papillary carcinoma in Hashimoto's thyroiditis. *Laryngoscope* 1997; 107(1): 95-100.

[42] Muzza M, Degl'Innocenti D, Colombo C, Perrino M, Ravasi E, Rossi S, Cirello V. The tight relationship between papillary thyroid cancer, autoimmunity and inflammation: clinical and molecular studies. *Clin Endocrinol (Oxf)* 2010; 72(5):702–08.

[43] Rhoden KJ, Unger K, Salvatore G, Yilmaz Y, Vovk V, Chiappetta G, Qumsiyeh MB, Rothstein JL, Fusco A, Santoro M, Zitzelsberger H, Tallini G. RET/papillary thyroid cancer rearrangement in nonneoplastic thyrocytes: follicular cells of Hashimoto's thyroiditis share low-level recombination events with a subset of papillary carcinoma. *J Clin Endocrinol Metab* 2006; 91(6):2414 –2423.

[44] Kim SK, Song KH, Limet SD et al. "Clinical and pathological features and the *BRAF*V600E mutation in patients with papillary thyroid carcinoma with and without concurrent Hashimoto thyroiditis," *Thyroid* 2009; 19(2):137–141.

[45] Larson SD, Jackson LN, Riall TS et al. Increased incidence of well-differentiated thyroid cancer associated with Hashimoto's thyroiditis and the role of the PI3k/Akt pathway. *J Am Coll Surg* 2007; 204(4):764-763.

[46] Anderson CE, Graham C, Herriot MM, Kamel HM, Salter DM. CD98 expression is decreased in papillary carcinoma of the thyroid and Hashimoto's thyroiditis. *Histopathology* 2009; 55(6), 683-686.

[47] Gürsoy A, Erdoğan MF. Ultrasonographic approach to thyroid nodules: state of art. *Thyroid international* 2012; 3:1-15.

[48] Mariotti S, Caturegli P, Piccolo P, Barbesino G, Pinchera A. Antithyroid peroxidase autoantibodies in thyroid diseases. *J Clin Endocrinol Metab* 1990; 71(3):661–669.

[49] Tunbridge WM, Evered DC, Hall R, Appleton D, Brewis M, Clark F, Evans JG, Young E, Bird T, Smith PA. The spectrum of thyroid disease in a community: the Whickham survey. *Clin Endocrinol (Oxf)* 1977; 7(6):481–493.

[50] Gutekunst R, Hafermann W, Mansky T, Scriba PC. Ultrasonography related to clinical and laboratory findings in lymphocytic thyroidits. *Acta Endocrinol (Copenh)* 1989; 121(1):129–135.

[51] Nordmeyer JP, Shafeh TA, Heckmann C. Thyroid sonography in autoimmune thyroiditis. A prospective study on 123 patients. *Acta Endocrinol (Copenh)* 1990; 122(3):391–395.

[52] Anderson L, Middleton WD, Teefey SA et al. Hashimoto thyroiditis: Part 1, sonographic analysis of the nodular form of Hashimoto thyroiditis. *Am J Roentgenol* 2010; 195(1):208-15 .

[53] Yeh HC, Futterweit W, Gilbert P. Micronodulation: ultrasonographic sign of Hashimoto thyroiditis. *J Ultrasound Med* 1996; 15(12):813–819.

[54] Kerr L. High-resolution thyroid ultrasound: the value of color Doppler. *Ultrasound Q* 1994; 12(1):21–44.

[55] Langer JE, Khan A, Nisenbaum HL, et al. Sonographic appearance of focal thyroiditis. *Am J Roentgenol* 2001; 176(3):751–754.

[56] Sostre S, Reyes MM. Sonographic diagnosis and grading of Hashimoto's thyroiditis. *J Endocrinol Invest* 1991; 14(2):115–121.

[57] Yildirim D, Gurses B, Gurpinar B, Eksi B, Colakoglu B, Kaur A. Nodule or Pseudonodule? Differentiation in Hashimoto's thyroiditis with sonoelastography. *The Journal of International Medical Research* 2011; 39(6): 2360 – 2369.

[58] Anderson L, Middleton WD, Teefey SA et al. Hashimoto thyroiditis: Part 2, sonographic analysis of benign and malignant nodules in patients with diffuse Hashimoto thyroiditis. *Am J Roentgenol* 2010; 195(1):216-23.

[59] Rago T, Santini F, Scutari M, Pinchera A, Vitti P. Elastography: new developments in ultrasound for predicting malignancy in thyroid nodules. *J Clin Endocrinol Metab* 2007; 92(8): 2917-2922.

[60] Rago T, Vitti P. Role of thyroid ultrasound in the diagnostic evaluation of thyroid nodules. *Best Pract Res Clin Endocrinol Metab* 2008; 22(6): 913–928.

[61] Kwak JY, Kim EK. Ultrasound elastography for thyroid nodules: recent advances. *Ultrasonography* 2014; 33(2):75-82.

[62] Carmela Asteria, Alessandra Giovanardi, Alessandro Pizzocaro, Luca Cozzaglio, Alberto Morabito, Francesco Somalvico, and Adele Zoppo. US-Elastography in the Differential Diagnosis of Benign and Malignant Thyroid Nodules. *Thyroid* 2008; 18(5): 523-531. doi:10.1089/thy.2007.0323..

[63] Rago T, Scutari M, Santini F et al. Real-time elastography: useful tool for refining the presurgical diagnosis in thyroid nodules with indeterminate or nondiagnostic cytology. *J Clin Endocrinol Metab* 2010; 95(12): 5274-5280.

[64] Magri F, Chytiris S, Capelli V, Gaiti M, Zerbini F, Carrara R, Malovini A, Rotondi M, Bellazzi R, Chiovato L. Comparison of elastographic Strain Index and thyroid Fine-Needle Aspiration Cytology in 631 Thyroid Nodules. *J Clin Endocrinol Metab*, December 2013; 98(12):4790 – 4797.

[65] Wang H, Brylka D, Sun LN, Lin YQ, Sui GQ, Gao J. Comparison of strain ratio with elastography score system in differentiating malignant from benign thyroid nodules. *Clinical Imaging* 2013; 37(1): 50–55.

[66] Magri F, Chytiris S, Capelli V, Alessi S, Nalon E, Rotondi M, Cassibba S, Calliada F, Chiovato L. Shear wave elastography in the diagnosis of thyroid nodules: feasibility in the case of coexistent chronic autoimmune Hashimoto's thyroiditis. *Clinical Endocrinology* 2012; 76(1): 137–141.

[67] Sahin M, Cakal E, Özbek M, Güngünes A, Arslan MS, Akkaymak ET, Ucan B, Ünsal IÖ, Bozkurt NC, Delibasi T. Elastography in the differential diagnosis of thyroid nodules in Hashimoto thyroiditis. *Med Oncol* 2014; 31(8): pp. 97 .

[68] Douglas PC, Faquin WC. Thyroid cytopathology. 2nd edition *Springer* 2010.

[69] Kumarasinghe MP, De Silva S. Pitfalls in cytological diagnosis of autoimmune thyroiditis. *Pathology* 1999; 31(1):1-7.

[70] MacDonald L, Yazdi HM. Fine needle aspiration biopsy of Hashimoto's thyroiditis. Sources of diagnostic error. *Acta Cytologica* 1999; 43(3) 400–406.

[71] Asa SL. My approach to oncocytic tumours of the thyroid. *J Clin Pathol* 2004; 57(3):225–232; doi: 11.1036/jcp.2003.008474.

[72] Baloch ZW, LiVolsi VA, Asa SL, Rosai J, Merino MJ, Randolph G, Vielh P, DeMay RM, Sidawy MK, Frable WJ. Diagnostic terminology and morphologic criteria for cytologic diagnosis of thyroid lesions: A synopsis of the National Cancer Institute Thyroid Fine-Needle Aspiration State of the Science Conference. *Diagn Cytopathol* 2008; 36(6): 425-437.

[73] McDougall IR. Management of Thyroid Cancer and Related Nodular Disease. *Springer* 2006.

[74] Ahn D, Heo SJ, Park JH, Kim JH, Sohn JH, Park JY, Park SK, Park J. Clinical relationship between Hashimoto's thyroiditis and papillary thyroid cancer. *Acta Oncol* 2011; 50(8):1228-34 doi: 10.3109/0284186X.2011.602109. .

[75] Di Pasquale M, Rothstein JL, Palazzo JP. Pathologic features of Hashimoto's-associated papillary thyroid carcinomas. *Human Pathology* 2001; 32(1):24–30.

[76] Sapino A, Papotti M, Macri L, Satolli MA, Bussolati G. Intranodal reactive endothelial hyperplasia in adenomatous goiter. *Histopathology* 26(5): 457-462, 1995.

[77] Siderova M, Hristozov K, Krasnaliev I, Softova E, Boeva E. Application of immunohistochemical markers in the differential diagnosis of thyroid tumors. *Acta Endocrinologica* 2013; 9(1): 41-52; doi: 10.4183/aeb.2013.41 .

[78] Kovacs RB, Földes J, Winkler G, Bodo M, Sapi Z. The investigation of galectin-3 in diseases of the thyroid gland. *Eur J Endocrinol* 2003; 149(5): 449-453.

[79] Prasad ML, Pellegata NS, Huang Y, Nagaraja NH, Chapelle A, Kloos RT. Galectin-3, fibronectin-1, CITED-1, $HBME_1$ and cytokeratin-19 immunohistochemistry is useful for the differential diagnosis of thyroid tumors. *Modern Pathology* 2005; 18(1): 48-57.

[80] Mataraci EA, Ozgüven BY, Kabukçuoglu F. Expression of cytokeratin 19, HBME-1 and galectin-3 in neoplastic and nonneoplastic thyroid lesions. *Pol J Pathol* 2012; 63(1): 58-64.

[81] Mase T, Funahashi H, Koshikawa T, Imai T, Nara Y, Tanaka Y, Nakao A. HBME-1 immunostaining in thyroid tumors especially in follicular neoplasm. *Endocr J* 2003; 50(2): 173-177.

[82] Papotti M, Volante M, Saggiorato E, Deandreis D, Veltri A, Orlandi F. Role of Galectin-3 immunodetection in the cytological diagnosis of thyroid cystic papillary carcinoma. *Eur J Endocrinol* 2002; 147(4): 515-521.

[83] Savin S, Cvejic D, Isic T, Paunovic I, Tatic S, Havelka M. Thyroid peroxidase and Galectin-3 immunostaining in differentiated thyroid carcinoma: diagnostic usefulness and clinicopathological correlation. *Hum Pathol* 2008; 39(11): 1656-1663.

[84] Ardito G, Revelli L, Boninsegna A, Sgambato A, Moschella F, Marzola MC, Giustozzi E, Avenia N, Castelli M, Rubello D. Immunohistochemical evaluation of inflammatory and proliferative markers in adjacent normal thyroid tissue in patients undergoing total

thyroidectomy: results of a preliminary study. *Journal of Experimental & Clinical Cancer Research* 2010, **29**:77 doi:10.1186/1756-9966-29-77.

[85] Cheung CC, Ezzat S, Freeman JL, Rosen IB, Asa SL. Immunohistochemical diagnosis of papillary thyroid carcinoma. *Mod Pathol* 2001; 14(4): 338-342.

[86] Tufano RP, Clayman G, Heller KS, Inabnet WB, Kebebew E, Shaha A, Steward DL, Tuttle RM for the American Thyroid Association Surgical Affairs Committee Writing Task Force. Management of recurrent/persistent nodal disease in patients with differentiated thyroid cancer: a critical review of the risks and benefits of surgical intervention versus active surveillance. *Thyroid* 2015; 25(1):15-27; doi: 10.1089/thy.2014.0098.

[87] Pacini F, Molinaro E, Castagna MG, Agate L, Elisei R, Ceccarelli C, Lippi F, Taddei D, Grasso L, Pinchera A. Recombinant human thyrotropin-stimulated serum thyroglobulin combined with neck ultrasonography has the highest sensitivity in monitoring differentiated thyroid carcinoma. *J Clin Endocrinol Metab* 2003; 88(8):3668–3673.

[88] Torlontano M, Crocetti U, Augello G, D'Aloiso L, Bonfitto N, VarrasoA, Dicembrino F, Modoni S, FruscianteV, DiGiorgio A, Bruno R, Filetti S, Trischitta. Comparative evaluation of recombinant human thyrotropin-stimulated thyroglobulin levels, 131I whole-body scintigraphy, and neck ultrasonography in the follow-up of patients with papillary thyroid microcarcinoma who have not undergone radioiodine therapy. *J Clin Endocrinol Metab* 2006; 91(1):60–63..

[89] Chung J-K, Park Y J, K im T Y et al. Clinical significance of elevated level of serum antithyroglobulin antibody in patients with differentiated thyroid cancer after thyroid ablation. *Clin Endocrinol* 2002; 57(2): 215-221.

[90] Rasmussen UF, Rasmussen AK. Autoimmunity in differentiated thyroid cancer: significance and related clinical problems. *Hormones* 2010; 9(2):109-117.

[91] Spencer CA. Clinical utility of Thyroglobulin Antibody (TgAb) measurements for patients with differentiated thyroid cancers (DTC). *J Clin Endocrinol Metab* 2011, 96(12):3615–3627.

[92] Larbre H, Schvartz C, Schneider N, et al. Positive antithyroglobulin antibodies in patients with differentiated thyroid carcinoma. What significance? *Ann Endocrinol (Paris)* 2000; 61(5): 422-427.

[93] Chiovato L, Latrofa F , Braverman LE, et al. Disappearance of humoral thyroid autoimmunity after complete removal of thyroid antigens. *Ann Intern Med* 2003; 139(5): 346-351.

[94] Kim WG, Yoon JH, Kim WB, Kim TY, Kim EY, Kim JM, Ryu JS, Gong G, Hong SJ, Shong YK. Change of serum antithyroglobulin antibody levels is useful for prediction of clinical recurrence in thyroglobulin-negative patients with differentiated thyroid carcinoma. *J Clin Endocrinol Metab* 2008; 93(12):4683–4689.

[95] Spencer A, Fatemi S. Thyroglobulin antibody (TgAb) methods – strengths, pitfalls and clinical utility for monitoring TgAb-positive patients with differentiated thyroid cancer. *Best Practice & Research Clinical Endocrinology & Metabolism* 2013; 27(5):701–712.

Index

A

D

H

I

N

O

P

Q

R

S

T

U

V

W

X

Y